The Collagen Type II Cure

Type II Cure

for

Arthritis

&

Heart Disease

CHICKEN STERNAL COLLAGEN TYPE II

THE NUTRI-MEDICAL REVELATION
OF THE MILLENIUM

by

Alex Duarte, O.D., Ph.D

Dedication

I dedicate this book to all those who have suffered with the terrible, relentless pain of arthritis. May you now find true relief with collagen type II.

Published October 1997, ISBN #1-891036-11-4

Table of Contents

Introduction

If you pinch your nose or wiggle it, bend your ear, extend your leg, comb your hair, exercise, and wrinkle your skin, all of this is possible because of connective tissue. The vast majority of connective tissue is called collagen.

Collagen is a proteinaceous substance, which is literally the glue that holds the body together. Collagen is found in many different tissues and it complexes with other substances to perform a variety of important functions. Collagen can be formed into strong, dense fibrils to make tendons that connect bone to muscle. It can be transformed into thin sheets to help form and keep skin cells connected. It also takes on a transparency to help form the front of the eye known as the cornea. When it comes to the skeleton of the human body, we find collagen helps knit bone and, thus, provides strength for this load bearing structure. Perhaps most important of all, collagen is the most ubiquitous part of cartilage which helps to provide some elasticity to joints and serves as a shock absorber therein. There are 14 known types of collagen. However, the most predominant is collagen type II and that is what this book is all about.

Collagen type II has a unique capacity to act as a skeleton for molecules known as proteoglycans. Think of collagen type II as the "super glue" that holds cartilage together. Because cartilage derived collagen type II complexes to important proteoglycans, it serves as a medicinal nutrient that can assist the body in recovering from a sundry of different diseases.

Collagen has been used externally for a number of years to reduce wrinkles and improve the natural beauty and healthy appearance of skin. It has also been systematically injected to remove wrinkles, and is part of an ever-growing number of superior skin care products that return youthful vitality and appearance to skin.

In addition to this cosmetic application, collagen type II has been shown to elicit through oral tolerance, a phenomenal immune response which literally has helped rheumatoid arthritis victims overcome this painful and progressive disease. It is also important to realize that only chicken sternal cartilage collagen type II has produced the remarkable amelioration of arthritic symptoms in medical research. This is probably due to the fact that the sternums (breastbones) of six- to eight-week-old chickens have the highest concentration of the collagen II proteoglycans, chondroitin sulfate A and glucosamine sulfate of any cartilage known.

Finally, because cartilage chicken sternal collagen type II complexes with these proteoglycans, such as chondroitin sulfate A and glucosamine sulfate, it has the ability to improve circulation and help restore damage to aging osteoarthritic joints. New research shows that collagen type II might even have an application in slowing or stopping the progression of myopia (near sightedness), breast implant poisoning, and Menier's disease. However, the greatest application of collagen type II as a therapeutic agent is far and away arthritis, and in particular osteo- and rheumatoid arthritis.

CHAPTER 1

The Story of Collagen Type II Begins with the Story of Cartilage

My discovery of the collagen type II cure began with a study of the substance that collagen type II comes from: Cartilage. In 1984, my father died of prostate cancer that had metastasized to the bone. Within one year after his death, some colleagues handed me several pounds of research on the most extraordinary discovery that cartilage could heal many diseases, including cancer. Motivating my efforts was my vow that I would search for an answer to this plague of the 21st century and not stop before I could find something that was effective and safe.

As I began to study the research on cartilage, I was amazed to find that it had very successful applications to many disorders. Cancer, arthritis, colitis, acne, psoriasis, ulcers, allergic dermatitis, cold sores, and even viral infections such as shingles responded favorably. How could so many diseases respond to one nutritional medicine? The answer came to me as a result of asking the question: What do all of these diseases have in common? The answer: "inflammation" and "pain". And, what is it in cartilage that addresses pain and inflammation? The answer: proteoglycans such as chondroitin sulfate A and glucosamine sulfate. And, what part of the cartilage holds these magnificent compounds? **Collagen Type II**. Finally I discovered, thanks to new research, the richest, purest source of these health-saving proteoglycans is young **Chicken Sternal Cartilage Collagen Type II**.

Thanks to the Chinese, we have an incredible, historical record of the use of cartilage as a natural medicament. Clinical studies show its efficacy against many different diseases. Today, we know the specific components of cartilage that have a wide range of healing potential. Before we get to the collagen type II component of cartilage and discover its tremendous healing power, we must first go back to China where for hundreds of years one of the most popular health tonics was shark fin soup. It is considered a "health tonic" delicacy even today.

One of the most prized parts of the shark is its fin, which is, of course, cartilage. The entire skeleton of a shark is cartilage, there are no bones in this fish. It is not unusual for the Chinese to pay anywhere from $10 or more for a bowl of life-giving shark fin soup. While the health promoting benefits of shark fin soup can be understood, the more extravagant claim of a powerful aphrodisiac needs to be tempered with an equal amount of doubt.

Six to eight percent of the gross weight of the shark's body is cartilage, and the cartilage of the shark in many biochemical ways is similar to the cartilage of cattle and humans. If we analyze this incredible medicinal substance, we find that cartilage is composed of collagen, fat and water, as much as 60% water. The collagen fraction is a combination of proteins interwoven electrostatically and biochemically with another type of substance called proteoglycans (mucopolysaccharides). Another name for proteoglycans is glycosaminoglycans. Basically, these are proteins and sugar molecules, hooked together in various ways, which contain other substances such as sulfur. Perhaps the most important proteoglycan substances, at least in terms of healing and reversing the disease known as arthritis, is glucosamine sulfate and chondroitin sulfate A, B and C. To the nonchemist, this sounds like a heap of foreign chemicals, however, let me assure you that each one of these substances plays a major role in terms of either initiating the healing response, reversing the arthritic degeneration of the joint, and/or dramatically reducing pain. If it is pain that has driven you to read these words, then you will have found the pot of gold at the end of the rainbow because it is within these substances that the powerful anti-inflammatory, pain-modulating power resides.

The healing potential of cartilage is really the healing potential of collagen type II and begins with the proteoglycans, or mucopolysaccharides as some scientists call them, such as chondroitin sulfate A and glucosamine sulfate. In order to appreciate the healing potential of collagen type II, we have to look at the research first conducted on cartilage. That forces us to go back to 1958, and the practice of Dr. John F. Prudden, a former Associate Professor of Surgery at the College of Physicians and Surgeons of Columbia University, Presbyterian Hospital in New York. Dr. Prudden developed a bovine (calf) cartilage extract that he made into a topical cream. He discovered that cartilage would dramatically accelerate wound healing following surgery. It proved highly effective, as a topical agent, in healing wounds such as varicose ulcers and post phlebitic ulcers.

Cartilage's anti-inflammatory properties were discovered serendipitously when Dr. Prudden treated a nonhealing ulcer on a leg of a man who also had psoriasis. After three days, both the ulcer and the psoriasis dramatically improved. Dr. Prudden correctly surmised that cartilage is a unique tissue and that, because it contains no blood vessels, there's something in cartilage that will resist the formation of blood vessels. This inhibition of new blood vessel formation is called antiangiogenesis. This substance must necessarily then decrease the inflammatory response and reduce pain.

The ability of cartilage to destroy tumors by prohibiting new blood vessel formation was not discovered or utilized in clinical trials until the beginning of the 1970s. However, Dr. G. J. Thorbecke, a Professor of Pathology at New York University Medical Center, found that in studies of mouse spleens, cartilage enhanced antibody production both in test tube and in the individual animals. Dr. Arthur Johnson, Professor and Chairman of Microbiology and Immunology at the University of Minnesota, Duluth School of Medicine, said that cartilage is a true biological response modifier in that it increases the ability of white cells to destroy bacteria and viruses, yet it decreases the inflammatory response.

In the meantime, the anecdotal list of therapeutic successes continued to grow geometrically in Dr. Prudden's practice. Beginning in 1974, Dr. Prudden reported the successful treatment of over 50 patients with osteoarthritis, mandibular alveolitis (dry socket), acne, poison oak and poison ivy, hemorrhoids, anal fissures, psoriasis, rheumatoid arthritis, ulcerative colitis, regional enteritis, and finally cancer. Realize, the healing elements of cartilage are locked up in that portion known as collagen type II, and chicken sternal cartilage collagen type II is the most effective.

Dr. Prudden first discovered the healing potential of the collagen type II proteoglycans of cartilage when he used it on wounds that would not heal on patients who were taking corticosteroids. It is a known side effect that medicines such as cortisone and prednisone inhibit the healing response. But in spite of the use of these drugs, cartilage would stimulate wound healing faster than the normal rate of healing, even in patients that were not taking these drugs. After several significant studies, Dr. Prudden teamed up with Dr. John Allen and, in 1965, conducted a study in which treated wounds were compared to control wounds. The overall increase in tensile strength resulting from the treatment was 42%, producing a difference that was highly significant. In addition, Dr. Prudden reconfirmed that collagen type II-rich cartilage has a powerful anti-inflammatory activity, along with its ability to improve and accelerate wound-healing.

In 60 chronically nonhealing open wounds, Dr. Prudden successfully generated a complete healing response in 59. This demonstrated the material was highly effective for humans as well as experimental animals.

Originally, the doctors were convinced the effective wound-healing ingredient in cartilage was a substance they termed "Poly-NAG", also known as polymeric-N-acetylglucosamine. Research indicated that, yes, Poly-NAG if isolated would greatly stimulate the healing of wounds. However, it is important to realize that Poly-NAG is one of those proteoglycans found in the collagen type II component of cartilage.

In a recent biochemical analysis, it was discovered that only chicken sternal cartilage contained exceptionally high levels of the anti-inflammatory proteoglycans. This analysis showed chondroitin sulfate A (CSA) is 14% of chicken sternal collagen type II, and the remarkable glucosamine sulfate is also 14% of chicken sternal collagen type II.

Collagen is not just one protein, there are over 14 different types of collagen, but the most prominent, the most important, the most medicinal, the one that has the greatest interaction with the proteoglycans just mentioned is collagen type II. Herein lies the fascinating story of the healing potential of cartilage itself. And more importantly, it must be understood that cartilage is an extremely difficult substance to digest and absorb. But when the cartilage matrix is broken up and the collagen type II is solubilized, there is a dramatic improvement in absorption and utilization of the healing components of this remarkable substance. Realize that as you are reading the success stories of cartilage, in essence you are reading the success stories of the major component of that cartilage, type II collagen with its associated proteoglycans. It is also important to realize, of all the various types of cartilage tested, the one that contained the highest level of anti-inflammatory proteoglycans, the one that showed the greatest healing potential was young chicken sternal cartilage. The six week old chicks beat out the sharks and all other sources of cartilage.

Perhaps the most debilitating and painful disease that commonly afflicts mankind is arthritis. Dr. Prudden reasoned that since the proteoglycan component of cartilage is the initial site of destruction in osteoarthritis; and since laboratory and clinical work has demonstrated an anti-inflammatory and wound healing effect of cartilage; and since cartilage provided the healthy biochemical components of cartilage (once again in the collagen type II fraction), it was reasonable to use cartilage as a therapeutic agent.

His assumptions were that a reconstruction of the affected cartilage would be achieved by furnishing the healthy biochemical components that could be utilized in the resynthesis of cartilage, providing he could reduce the inflammation. Dr. Prudden's reasoning was sound since Dr. A. J. Bollet had shown, in 1968, that collagen type II rich cartilage extracts stimulate protein and chondroitin sulfate synthesis.[1] Dr. Prudden went on to show large oral doses of cartilage were effective in the treatment of arthritis.

Realize cartilage, be it cows (bovine) cartilage or shark cartilage, is difficult to digest. It must be ground to about a 200-mesh particle size to have a chance of even partial absorption. By hydrolyzing the cartilage and taking the fraction that is holding the anti-inflammatory proteoglycans known as collagen type II, you have now put the cartilage components into a much more absorbable, effective, utilizable form known as collagen type II.

This is very significant when one considers that the standard treatment with Non-Steroidal Anti-Inflammatory Drugs (NSAIDS) has a dismal failure rate and does not stop the progression of the disease. These drugs temporarily reduce the inflammation, pain, and suffering but ultimately fail and hasten destruction of the joint.

Please understand cartilage is difficult to absorb, requiring 12 (750 milligrams) capsules daily to get a response. Also, shark cartilage is high in calcium and can be constipating. Soluble collagen type II is more absorbable, requiring less volume to

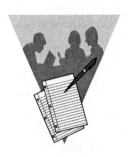

be consumed in order to get an equivalent response. Collagen type II does not have a lot of minerals, it is not constipating, and ounce for ounce contains more of those joint saving, pain killing proteoglycans. This makes collagen type II not only more therapeutically effective but also more cost effective. Also it has no offensive odor.

Recently, BioCell Technology, a California based company, has made an incredible technological breakthrough in delicately extracting bioactive chicken sternal collagen type II. BioCell Technology holds a patent pending on this extraordinary process that preserves the joint-saving, arthritis fighting, soluble proteoglycans.

Today there are several companies that sell this high quality, highly purified chicken sternal collagen type II. It is my hope that many others will carry this incredible product in the future. However, in order to illustrate the greater efficacy of chicken sternal collagen type II versus cartilage, note the following testimonial of a Ms. Betty S. from Kingman, Arizona.

Testimonials from People Taking Chicken Sternal Type II Collagen

To Whom It May Concern,

A few weeks ago I decided to try Immu Cell™ after having received an article on it. My left hip was giving me problems. I had trouble getting out of bed in the morning. I was taking quite a bit of Tylenol. Since taking ImmuCell™ after three plus weeks I have no problem getting up in the morning and taking my capsules. Within one hour the little ache I have is gone. This has all happened on three capsules. Sure beats surgery!

Thank you, Betty S., Kingman, Arizona   (testimony on file)

Also, don't be fooled into thinking Knox Gelatin is the same as collagen type II. Note the following testimonials:

I heard about the Harvard Study sometime ago and was using Knox Unflavored Gelatin and orange juice for my knee pain. I had good results as long as I would take the gelatin twice a day. It was very inconvenient. When I read about the ImmuCell™, I decided to try it. I figured it would cost about the same and be a whole lot easier to swallow. Not only was it more convenient, it seems to be far more effective and I only take it once a day as the bottle recommends.

Ronald A. W. Virginia Beach,Virginia   (testimony on file)

I am a Certified Nutritional Consultant and work with people who are arthritic and they also are having good results.

North Carolina   (testimony on file)

I have been taking ImmuCell™ on the recommendation of my Nutritional Consultant for a little over a month and find it effective at relieving pain in my hands and shoulder.

Grover C. B., Suffolk,Virginia   (testimony on file)

About a year ago, I started having trouble with my knees. It became very painful to go up stairs. I had relief, though, whenever I was consistent in taking Knox Unflavored Gelatin and orange juice. My husband heard about ImmuCell™ and switched us over to it mainly for convenience. I was reluctant at first but have found that not only is it more convenient, it

is more effective. Whenever I was not consistent in taking Knox Unflavored Gelatin and orange juice twice a day, I suffered. With the ImmuCell™, I only have to take it once a day and if I miss a day, I still have no pain. Thank you!

Linda W. Virginia Beach, Virginia　　　　　(testimony on file)

I have been using CellRenew™ for $2\frac{1}{2}$ months and have noticed a significant improvement in the chronic joint pain I had been experiencing. I have suffered from the pain of arthritic immobility of one of my fingers for several years. The bonus is the complete remission of pain in the other joints as well. I am so confident that this product has been dramatically instrumental in the improvement of my condition, that I know it will continue to be my daily routine. Because I have always been very resistant to taking painkillers, CellRenew™ has been nothing short of a blessing.

Mrs. Z.E., Tucson, AZ　　　　　(testimony on file)

The almost constant pain and increasing immobility in my shoulders and hands that I suffered with for many years is now reversed and continues to improve with regular use of CellRenew™. It took several months to realize initial relief, but now I notice improvement almost every day. Thank you for making me aware that I no longer have to suffer from my symptoms of the side effects of drug therapy.

Mrs. G.T., Pittsburgh, PA　　　　　(testimony on file)

Pain control and reduction of inflammation is what collagen type II and its associated mucopolysaccharides are all about.

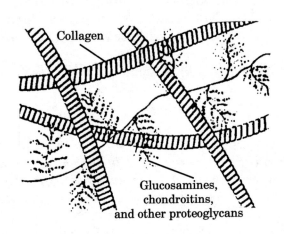

Electron micrograph shown at an elargement of 61,000 diameters. Showing the fibrils (rod-like aggregates) of the collagen protein. Note the dark stained collapsed masses of giant molecular mucopolysaccharides also known as proteoglycans. These proteoglycans include glucosamine, chondroitin, cartilage matrix glycoprotein, and other proteoglycans that hold water and give strength to cartilage.

CHAPTER 2

Chicken Sternal Collagen Type II and Arthritis

It may begin with stiffness in your knees; having worked in the garden the day before, you wake up with an ache or an excruciating pain in the lower back. Your fingers are stiff, hard to move and painful, you can't open that jar of jam like you used to. Maybe you're now having trouble walking, let alone jogging, simply because it hurts too much. That morning stiffness now requires two aspirin instead of one. Finally, the pain drives you to your physician for prescription medication, and while you don't like the idea of some of the side effects, you can't tolerate the hurt. You have to do something about it.

More than 50 million Americans, one in every seven, suffer from this disease known as arthritis. Yet, almost everyone past the age of fifty has some signs of it, and you don't have to look very hard to find them. Arthritis has become the leading cause of disability in our population and a lot of it has to do with our sedentary lifestyle. With the industrial revolution, our ancestors experienced revolutionary work changes. It used to be that people would simply grow their food or make what they needed, but because of industrialization people began to do one job, earn a wage, and make a living quite differently from the way their ancestors did. They no longer had to grow their own food, work in the fields, or make their own furniture. Jobs became specialized, automation led to less physical exertion in order to perform each task. And because most people no longer had to exert their bodies to obtain food, life became leisurely even though the psychological stresses became greater.

Today, people simply live longer than their ancestors did, and our bodies and joints have had to endure longer years. As a result they experience an increase in degenerative disease, including arthritis. However, arthritis is a very unique degenerative disease because it is a disease of the joints. It is related to the traumatic overuse or underuse of the joints as well as infection, unique immunity, aging, and genetics.

Dietary factors play a significant role in arthritis. Perhaps consumption of too many calories alone is a leading 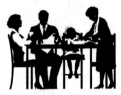 contributing factor because of obesity. With increasing age, we now know that proper, scientifically designed nutrition can prevent, delay, even effectively treat this painful disease that makes some people hurt all the time.

Interestingly enough, it's not the common cold or the flu bug, but rather joint pain that is the leading cause of lost time from work in our society today. Although many of the complications of joints are labeled arthritis, the true definition of arthritis is: "inflammation of a joint." Technically, arthritis is not just one disease because the inflammation in the joint can be caused by a number of factors, as I have already stated. Arthritis, rather, is a group of diseases that have common symptoms such as pain, inflammation and loss of movement. Actually, there are more than a hundred diseases that afflict the joints. The most common is a type of arthritis called osteoarthritis. The second most common type of arthritis relates to an immune reaction to the body itself, particularly to a type of collagen in the cartilage called collagen type II. While the cause of rheumatoid arthritis is totally different than that of osteoarthritis, the end result is the same: pain, inflammation, and more pain.

This book is going to explore a collagen type II therapy that can dramatically change your life if you suffer from arthritis. Not only because it is going to attack the very cause of the disease, but it is going to change that one simple, unavoidable, terrible, and paralyzing part of this disorder called "pain."[2]

Yes, nature has a cure. Nature has a remedy. When scientifically applied, it goes beyond the Motrin®, Advil®, or Tylenol®. And certainly we thank our creator for these wonderful pain relievers and for some of the more powerful painkillers like the nonsteroidal anti-inflammatories (NSAIDS). Yet, we now know that some of these painkillers, like the NSAIDS, have the ability to speed up the progression of arthritis. Let's take a moment to thank those wonderful surgeons who have spent the better part of their earlier years in intense study and training to relieve the pain of mankind through their masterful, operative abilities. We should look upon surgery as, yes, a blessing and certainly indicated for some, but always as a last resort only after all other approaches have failed.

What you will be surprised to learn in the following pages is that studies have already been completed to show, both in animal and human trials, that wonderful, natural products like collagen type II and its related proteoglycans can ameliorate this disease for the rest of your life. Why turn to an alternative? Why seek out another method if aspirin, NSAIDS, or surgery can do the job? The answer is simple. Aspirin can burn a hole in your stomach. NSAIDS can kill you by causing occult bleeding in the stomach and other parts of the gastrointestinal area. Surgery is painful, expensive, and not permanent. Finally, ten years after replacement, the joint will begin to fail again requiring a possible second surgery. Don't forget that many physicians still will tell their patients, "There's nothing more that can be done, except these procedures."

However, I contend that a great deal more can be done and that these natural therapies now have a scientific basis in the medical and health food applications. If you as an individual suffer from this hideous disease, then you have the right to choose a nontoxic, natural, effective approach. My job as the harbinger of this philosophy is to prove to you, to show to you, to help you understand that you have options that will work. I offer you a challenge and a promise. The challenge is to read the following pages completely through to the end of this book. If you are convinced enough to try the collagen type II cure, it is my personal promise that you will have the greatest chance of recovering from the pain and destruction of this disease.

CHAPTER 3

Osteoarthritis

Osteoarthritis is also known as degenerative joint disease. It is simply the most common form of arthritis. It results from the systematic loss of cartilage and then bone tissue in the joints. It typically plagues the elderly and is characterized by the protective cartilage at the ends of the bones wearing away. The cartilage is not replaced as fast as it is torn down, leading to the inner surfaces of the bone becoming exposed to each other and rubbing against one another. In some cases, bone spurs develop at the edges of the joints. As you can imagine, this is extremely painful. These spurs can cause damage to muscles, nerves, and result in deformity and difficulty in movement.

The precise cause of osteoarthritis is not yet known, but some very learned authorities speculate that it may result from a genetic predisposition to the disease, and certainly undue stress on particular joints, a broken or injured bone or joint, and dietary deficiencies endured over a period of years. Other authorities feel that it is simply a part of the aging process, but this theory is no longer popular. In rare cases, it can come on misuse or overuse of anabolic steroids used by some athletes to improve their physical performance. In other cases, where a disease state requires the use of medicines like prednisone, a cortico-steroid, osteoarthritis might also

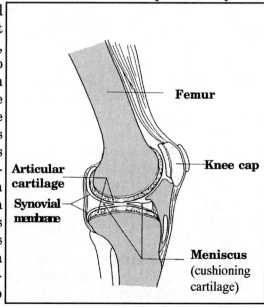

Femur

Knee cap

Articular cartilage

Synovial membrane

Meniscus (cushioning cartilage)

occur. Whatever the cause, the severity varies in every case and in some it may simply mean pain and stiffness in certain joints while others may have knarled, deformed joints and painful muscle inflammation to the point that any movement is restricted.

The word osteoarthritis comes from the Greek translation of the word osteo, which means of the bone, and arthro, which means joint. The ending of the word, itis, simply means inflammation, but bone and joint inflammation may vary from one type of arthritis to another. In osteoarthritis there is not the same degree of inflammation that occurs with rheumatoid arthritis for instance. Yet, there is still considerable pain associated with this form of the disease.

Osteoarthritis affects the cartilage, between the bones, called articular cartilage. This is a unique structure and nature has provided it with an extremely low coefficient of friction. Simply put, it's more slippery than ice. Just like ice, it has a bluish-white color. Who hasn't seen the gristle on the end of a chicken drumstick? And, of course, some of us have eaten it. This is the articular cartilage. However, this is too simple an explanation of what osteoarthritis is, because it affects the ends of the bone where the cartilage is attached as well as the cartilage itself. It also has degenerative problems associated with the capsule that surrounds the joint and the muscles that are adjacent to the joint as well as the fluid within the joint.

However, the disease process begins in the cartilage. Interestingly enough, about 65 to 80% of the cartilage is 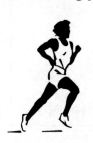 water. This helps to reduce the friction caused by one bone rubbing against another. Every time you walk, run, jump or get out of bed, this cartilage blunts the trauma of your weight bearing on the joint. I've always thought of cartilage as the springs of the body; the shock absorbers that help keep us moving and reduce trauma. The fluid that circulates between the articular cartilage, the bones themselves, and the membranes surrounding the cartilage (called the synovial membrane) is called the synovial fluid. This is a dynamic and important part of the joint. It carries nutrients into the cartilage because the healthy, normal joints have no blood vessels. The joint relies on a diffusion of nutrients from distant capillary beds and an exchange of waste material through the synovial fluid and cartilage.

Thus, every time you walk and your weight bears on the joint, specifically on the cartilage, the synovial fluid is squeezed out of the cartilage and circulates. Therefore, movement and exercise actually helps remove waste and brings in the nutrients needed for the cartilage and synovial fluid to remain healthy. Then, as you pick up your leg and remove the weight from the joint, the synovial fluid runs back into the cartilage, thus, the fluid moves in and out thanks to the force of exertion.

One of the beginning problems associated with this osteoarthritic disease is that the cartilage tends to dry out. This dramatically reduces its ability to act as a shock absorber, which allows greater trauma to the cartilage, and to the bones underneath the cartilage. A part of the cartilage responsible for regeneration begins to break down long before symptoms are actually experienced, and as the disease progresses the cartilage begins to soften and finally crack. When the cartilage begins to disintegrate, bone rubs on bone and this creates an excruciating type of pain. Bone deformities then result in ever increasing degrees of inflammation.

It is interesting to note that osteoarthritis attacks particular joints that are more likely to disintegrate and be affected than others. The most common osteoarthritic joints are the knees, hips, lower back, neck, fingers, and in some cases the joints in the feet as well. One of the distinguishing characteristics between osteoarthritis and rheumatoid arthritis is that in osteoarthritis usually one side is afflicted while the other is not, at least in the beginning stages of the disease. Thus, one knee may be very painful and the other will only ache a slight amount. Whereas, one hip may be much more painful than the other.

During the course of this disease, the body tries to fight back. New cartilage and new bone might be laid down. This is the body's way of compensating for what has already been lost. However, this new cartilage cannot replace what is lost and the new bone might be in a particular position that creates more pain and inflammation. Thus, these efforts, while valiant, are simply not adequate. The cartilage becomes pitted, the bones become fragmented and even small pieces of bone can float in the synovial fluid, creating additional pain and inflammation.

One of the symptoms of this disease is known as crepitus, which is simply a crackling sound that occurs as the joint is moved. It is most commonly heard in the knee and is a result of the joints rubbing together. People who suffer with arthritis call this the 'creaking knee' and friends, as well as relatives, can hear this disquieting sound. When your physician hears it, he knows he is looking at an advanced stage of the disorder.

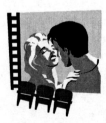 For most arthritics pain does not accompany this sound, but it is a little frightening. A much more motion-limiting phenomenon of osteoarthritic's joints is the locking up of the joint after periods of inactivity, perhaps sitting in the movie theater too long or riding in a car for an extended period of time. In the early stages of the disease, stiffness is only briefly experienced and can usually be rubbed out or walked out as movement occurs. However, the disease worsens and there is a time when permanent loss of range of motion occurs even after exercise or continual motion. The body is simply trying to stop any movement that is, at this point and time, creating a great deal of tissue damage. In most instances, by this time, surgery is indicated.

Another aspect of this disease, as with rheumatoid arthritis, is deformity and joint enlargement. Bone spurs actually limit the range of motion of the joint, and finally, fluid starts to accumulate in the joint. It's not uncommon for a rheumatologist to remove over four ounces of fluid from a single inflamed and swollen joint. Many arthritics know this as 'water on the knee'.

In osteoarthritis the initial lesions occur in the articular cartilage. However, some researchers believe that the fluid within the joint itself, known as the synovial fluid, begins to change its composition, which assists in the breakdown in the cartilage. The ends of the bones, known as *subchondral bone*, also can participate in the degeneration. The capsule that surrounds the joint and the synovial membrane will also make its contribution, as I will demonstrate later. Remember that normal, healthy cartilage contains a great deal of water, upwards of 80%, and the proteoglycans are also known as glycosaminoglycans or mucopolysaccharides. The unique construction of the cartilage allows for tremendous reduction in friction between the subchondral bone and allows for smooth and easy movement. Some scientists claim that cartilage is over eight times more slippery than ice.

In order to understand how this disease can be controlled and even reversed, it's important to understand its cause. Osteoarthritis is divided into two types: primary and secondary. The primary form of the disease is by far the most common and is considered to be a progressive type of degeneration. Normally, individuals past the age of 40 are most likely to incur this type of osteoarthritis. Furthermore, the disease tends to affect the weight bearing joints such as the hips, lower back, neck, and, of course, the knees.

Primary osteoarthritis can occur more frequently with individuals who show a family history of the disease. It also occurs considerably more often in people that are obese. Additionally, trauma to the joint caused by excessive loads or loads that are endured over a long period of time can cause enough trauma to initiate the disease. Remember that the initial degeneration is in the cartilage itself. Thus, the trauma induced by carrying excessive weight over a period of time will damage the cartilage. Realize that the knees, hips, lower back, the weight bearing joints of the body are handling over eight times a person's body weight depending on the type of movement encountered. If a person is carrying excessive amounts of weight and there is a lack of cartilage supporting nutrients or maybe even circulation problems which compromise the health of the cartilage in the joint, then it's easy to see that around the age of 40 or 45 there can be initial degeneration of the cartilage. Researchers have determined that obese, middle-aged women are the most susceptible to osteoarthritis. Thus, maintaining proper body weight can be one of the healthiest things you can do, not only for your heart and blood pressure, but also your joints.

Researchers have determined that the millions of people that are suffering with osteoarthritis are doing so with the help of their genes. Scientists have actually isolated the defective DNA, on the twelfth chromosome that's associated with this form of arthritis.[3]

Secondary osteoarthritis is different in that it appears before the age of 40 and is clearly a disease caused by injury to the joint. This injury can be from poor nutrition, chronic trauma, and even infection. Sometimes surgical procedures and secondary injuries to joints aggravate the disease. Early injury to the knee joint, for instance, can cause a permanent stretching of ligaments and tendons, allowing for a loose joint to occur. As this loss of connective tissue strength occurs, there is greater impact on cartilage and other joint tissues as a result of running, skiing, jumping, or other activity that over time provides an additive trauma to the joint.

Repetitive movement that occurs over time can cause chronic trauma to the joint. The professional dancer that uses the joint in a more repetitive way than the average person can sustain small injuries that over time will lead to damage of the joint. Professional baseball, football, and hockey players are common candidates for joint trauma. Certain jobs can also provide greater stresses and strains on weight bearing joints. It has been demonstrated that with the passage of time, the mucopolysaccharide portion of the joint, that portion that holds the water in the cartilage, changes. It shifts from a predominance of what scientists call chondroitin-4-sulfate to a greater amount of a juvenile type of cartilage called keratin-sulfate. Scientists such as Dr. John F. Prudden, who initially researched the phenomenal medicinal values of therapeutic cartilage, showed that the mucopolysaccharide component of the cartilage, the component that is intertwined with collagen type II, apparently shows the initial damage in osteoarthritis. Both laboratory and clinical research has shown an anti-inflammatory effect and wound-healing effect of orally ingested cartilage. This is apparently because cartilage provides the healthy biochemical components such as collagen type II, which contains a natural anti-inflammatory, chondroitin sulfate A. In this book, we will examine the almost miraculous healing properties of collagen type II as the primary component of cartilage.

Men tend to engage in more strenuous and sometimes more traumatic activity than women do, accounting for a greater incidence of osteoarthritis up to the age of 45. Approximately two percent of the population suffer with this disease under the age of 45. Past the age of 45 up to about age 65, the rise in the incidence of osteoarthritis is sudden, going to 30%. Past the age of 65, statistics show that over 80% will suffer with the disease.[4]

When the population of osteoarthritis sufferers gets past the age of 55, women display the disease twice as often as men do.

Note the following diagram and observe that a normal, healthy joint has healthy, smooth, articular cartilage that is bathed in a nourishing, waste removing synovial fluid, produced by a healthy, normal synovial membrane. All of this is encapsulated in a joint capsule. In the osteoarthritic joint there is considerable damage, pitting, and flaking of the articular cartilage that results in damage and pitting to the subchondral bone.

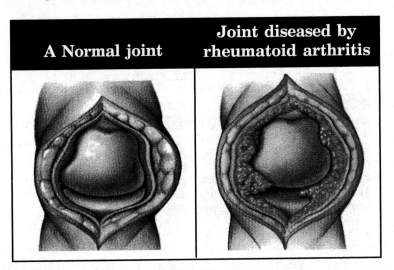

A Normal joint

Joint diseased by rheumatoid arthritis

This, in turn, leads to an attempt by the body to compensate for the damage by producing weakened cartilage and bone spurs.

Finally, bone will rub on bone and generate the enormous pain and loss of range of motion of osteoarthritis. Eventually, in the later stages, deformity and joint enlargement with inflammation occurs, as well as water on the knee. Joint cracking known as *crepitus* occurs and the patient feels a crunching feeling emanating from the joint when the patient starts to walk or move the leg. Most of the time this is the knee joint. It can occur in the hip, but it most often strikes the knees creating the creaking that can be heard from across a room.

The Key to Cartilage Health is Collagen Type II

Collagen type II is made from protein and forms a large part of the cartilage matrix. In fact, it is collagen that is responsible for the various components of cartilage being held together. Remember that cartilage is a combination of water, collagen, and proteoglycans called mucopolysaccharides, as well as a small amount of fat. This entire complex is known as the cartilage matrix. If the cartilage matrix is strong and healthy, it is extremely resistant to trauma, disease, or age related diseases. Collagen provides some elasticity to cartilage giving it a tremendous ability to absorb shock. The mucopolysaccharide fraction is composed of very large molecules. Muco means proteins and polysaccharide means many sugars. Thus, the mucopolysaccharides are a combination of protein and sugars. THE MUCO-POLYSACCHARIDES ARE INTER-WOVEN THROUGH AND AROUND COLLAGEN. THE MUCOPOLYSACCHARIDE IS AN INTRICATE PART OF THIS MESHWORK MATRIX AND ITS PRIMARY JOB IS TO HOLD WATER. This helps to make cartilage resilient and allows it to stretch back to a normal position once it has been compressed during running, walking, and other activity.

Throughout the collagen type II mucopolysaccharide matrix there are cartilage-producing cells called chondrocytes. These small cells produce new collagen and new mucopolysaccharide molecules making sure there is replacement of these structures when they are lost. Chondrocytes also produce an enzyme that degrades and disposes of old collagen and mucopolysaccharide molecules that have lived past their usefulness.

When Things Go Wrong

One of the problems in osteoarthritis is that the chondrocytes no longer regulate the correct proportion of collagen to mucopolysaccharide to water. In an effort to restore normal structural integrity, more chondrocytes are produced. This, in turn, generates greater amounts of collagen and mucopolysaccharides as well as fluid that, unfortunately, wash these materials out of the system. With time this results in a smaller amount of the structural components of the cartilage. Collagen type II fibers in the cartilage can become smaller. The once very dense matrix of collagen type II and mucopolysaccharides is now compromised with the result of loss of mucopolysaccharides and the water holding ability of the cartilage. Dry cartilage becomes damaged easily, showing small holes and cracks. This, in turn, produces a fast wearing cartilage.

This is only part of the problem. The chondrocytes may start producing greater levels of collagen dissolving enzymes, and as the collagen type II, the glue, the nucleus of the cartilage is destroyed, so then is the cartilage. The enzymes also have a dissolving effect on the mucopolysaccharides and so they are an ever-increasing problem in the destruction of the joint. Now, without healthy cartilage to cushion them, the bones begin to show signs of wear which leads to rough, bumpy surfaces with their own fractures and degeneration.

Certain dietary factors may play a significant role in the progression of this disease. For instance, a diet that is rich in saturated omega-6 fats produces a prevalence of inflammatory prostaglandins which helps elevate the level of inflammation within the joints. A diet that is lacking the omega-3 fats can lead to production of less viscous, more watery, synovial fluid, one that is not as healthy and one that cannot nourish the cartilage and other structures within the joint itself. Therefore, eat a diet rich in omega-3 fats.

Alcoholism, which depletes the body's reserves of magnesium and other nutrients, can lead to a faster progression of osteoarthritis; and certainly infection, along with chronic trauma to the joint, speeds up the degeneration process. Also, a diet that is too rich in sugar will purge calcium from the body and weaken bone structures, allowing for a faster osteoarthritic degeneration. Certain minerals such as manganese, copper, iron, calcium, magnesium, and boron are crucial to the strength and resistance of bone to early degeneration. Furthermore, liver disease that can be caused from alcoholism or hepatitis, which is caused by virus infections, can compromise the growth hormones and enzymes that are necessary for proper cartilage and bone formation, thus allowing a faster degeneration of the cartilage matrix.

Finally, as the disease progresses and the lining of the joint, the synovial membrane, becomes more and more inflamed, it is less able to produce the most important fluid, the synovial fluid, that nourishes the cartilage and removes the waste. This lubricating substance, if compromised, becomes unable to reduce friction and it loses its ability to lubricate. The end result of the ailing joint is extreme pain due to swelling. This may, in fact, lead the patient to take pain killing drugs such as nonsteroidal anti-inflammatories or even more powerful corticosteroid drugs like prednisone. In both instances, these types of drugs speed up the osteoarthritic condition and actually hasten the destruction of the joint.

But take heart, because now with scientific research showing us the way, we see that by ingesting the various components of cartilage, particularly the primary component, collagen type II, we may be able to not only reduce the terrible pain of this disease, the inflammation, but also reverse its destructive potential. We know that collagen type II and the mucopolysaccharides intertwined within collagen type II, the proteoglycans known as glucosamines and chondroitins, can produce an enormous protective pharmiconutrient restoration of cartilage and the joint itself. Let's now take a closer look at these components of cartilage as they relate to osteoarthritis.

Glucosamine: The Key To Strong Cartilage and Other Connective Tissue

One of the important ingredients in tendons and in the synovial fluid of the joint is hyaluronic acid. It also serves as the backbone of the proteoglycans, those water loving mucopolysaccharides that keep the cartilage an effective cushion when walking, jogging, running, and engaging in other movement.

Glucosamine, found within collagen type II, is the pivotal compound in connective tissue repair and production. It turns out that glucose can be bypassed in the production of glucosamine as a rate-limiting step. Over 30 years of research has shown that glucosamine is the precursor for the proteoglycan production (glucosaminoglycans) and is the preferred substrate (building block) for these compounds, including chondroitin sulfate, hyaluronic acid and collagen type II itself.

In test tube cultures, cartilage and connective tissue cells were found to produce significantly higher amounts of hyaluronic acid and more CSA, collagen type II, and matrix proteins when glucosamine was added. Glucosamine added to human cartilage improved its mechanical properties and most important of all, glucosamine increased proteoglycan production by 170% in cultured connective tissue cells. All other proteoglycans were inefficient in accomplishing this task.

Low doses, that is to say normal doses, physiological doses, when taken by animals increased cartilage synthesis by 10%, which is an enormous amount. THIS INDICATES THAT GLUCOSAMINE NOT ONLY PROTECTS CARTILAGE, IT REBUILDS AND STIMULATES THE PRODUCTION OF CARTILAGE.

One study showed over 70% absorption of glucosamine while still other studies have shown up to 95% absorption in animal and human trials. As an interesting side note, 30% of orally ingested glucosamine is stored in muscles for long periods of time to be used as the body needs it. Daily consumption of glucosamine was found to raise the tissue levels better than intravenous administration. Glucosamine is nontoxic and oral doses as high as 8 grams for every 2.2 pounds of body weight have not caused any problems even after months of dosing. Let's take a close look at some of the human studies regarding glucosamine as a powerful alleviator of pain and potent regenerator of cartilage tissue.

The study I will describe now was actually conducted in Portugal and sponsored by the University of Pavia, in Pavia, Italy. It included 252 doctors throughout Portugal who were to assess the effectiveness and tolerability of oral glucosamine sulfate in the treatment of arthrosis. Patients received 2 capsules, 250 milligrams each, three times daily for a total of 1.5 grams. The study lasted for a period of 14 days and the results of 1,208 patients were assessed.

The assessment involved the degree of pain at rest, on standing and on exercise. Limited active and passive movements were also analyzed. The ratings that were to be used by the doctors in determining success were: good, sufficient and insufficient.

At the time the study ended 1,183 patients could be rated considering the normal number of dropouts. The doctors objectively rated the therapeutic results as good in 694 (58.7%) of the patients, the rating of sufficient was given to 426 (36%) of the patients and insufficient results were reported in only 63 (5.3%) patients.[5]

The authors of the study, Angelo A. Bignamini, Macario Joao Tapadinhas and Italo Croce Riva, concluded that these results were significantly better than of those obtained with previous, conventional, drug type of therapies in the same patients. Sex, age, localization of the arthritis, concomitant illnesses, as well as concomitant treatment for those illnesses did not influence the frequency of responders to the treatment. This simply means that if patients were taking heart medicines or medicines for ulcers or other types of medications, oral glucosamine had no influence on those other drugs or therapies.

Oral glucosamine was fully tolerated by 86% of the patients, a far larger proportion than with any other conventional drug treatment. Onset of improvement of symptoms was extremely fast and the improvement obtained even after the medicines were discontinued after 14 days, lasted for a period of six to 12 weeks following the end of treatment.

As an interesting side note of the study, approximately 112 patients of the study who did not respond to previous types of conventional drug therapies benefited tremendously from the glucosamine administration. This is extremely exciting in that it demonstrates glucosamine is a very powerful modulator of pain and inflammation.

Note the following pain score graph. Remember collagen type II contains a very high concentration of glucosamine in addition to other important joint protecting proteoglycans.

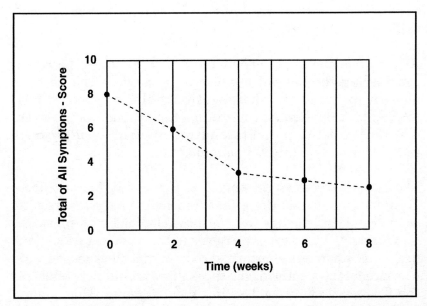

[Modified from: Tapadinhas, M.J., Rivera, I.C., and Bignamini, A. A., "Oral Glucosamine Sulphate in the Management of Arthrosis: Report on a Multicenter Open Investigation in Portugal." Pharmatherapeutica 3(3): 157-168, 1982.]

If we take a close look at the graph, we see that the total of all symptoms score, which included range of motion, mobility, and reduction of pain showed a dramatic response to orally ingested glucosamine in a short period of time, with the majority of the response being around four weeks. The authors themselves concluded that the oral treatment with glucosamine manages most arthritis patients to FULL OR PARTIAL RECOVERY, whatever the location of their arthrosis and in spite of concomitant illness or treatments.

The only slight complication that arose was that some patients that were on diuretics (which are designed to waste water) did not have the proper response to the diuretics. Glucosamine holds water and the diuretic medication dose had to be adjusted. This is a very small price to pay for loss of pain, increased range of motion, and dramatic improvement in quality of life.

Look at the date that this study was conducted, 1982. You would have thought that every doctor in the world would have rushed to use glucosamine sulfate in the management of arthritis, but such was not the case. Pharmaceutical companies have big bills, big prices, and big profits. None of these fall into the category of a natural, nontoxic, orally ingested collagen type II derived product called glucosamine. If we recall the analysis of collagen type II we remember that the glucosamine fraction is 14%, so 3 to 6 grams of collagen type II daily will give you more than enough proteoglycans to match the dosage that is conventionally used in this type of study and in clinical settings.

What is so interesting is that the next study we'll consider was conducted a year earlier. It is amazing to me that the medical profession has not embraced this incredible technology until just recently. The next study, conducted in 1981, in Parma, Italy, involved 30 patients with osteoarthritis. Two groups of inpatients received either a placebo daily, for seven days, or injection of glucosamine sulfate (400 milligrams). Whereas during the two following weeks the patients receiving glucosamine had oral glucosamine capsules (1.5 grams daily) and another group had a placebo.

The efficacy of the treatment was determined by a pain scoring system that involved active and passive movements, as well as limitation of the movement itself before and after the 7- and 21-day treatment periods. The patients were also questioned daily for any intolerance of the symptoms and standard blood work and urinalysis were conducted before and after the treatment.

During the initial treatments, each symptom significantly improved but to a faster and greater extent in the group treated with glucosamine. During the maintenance period a further improvement was recorded in patients treated with glucosamine, whereas those on placebo had symptom scores actually increase almost to the pretreatment level. This was considered the major difference between the control placebo and the therapeutic glucosamine. The tolerance for the glucosamine was excellent and no drug complaints were recorded. The authors concluded their study by stating that the glucosamine should be considered the basic therapy for primary and secondary degenerative osteoarthritis.

We know, and it has been shown, that glucosamine is the primary pivotal substrate that stimulates proteoglycan biosynthesis, inhibits the degeneration of proteoglycans in cartilage and actually rebuilds experimentally damaged cartilage. Note the following chart and observe there was a decrease in the overall symptom score of 58% during the initial injection of glucosamine and a further 13% with oral maintenance therapy.[6] This decrease was significantly larger than that measured during the treatment with placebo. The limited improvement recorded during the initial treatment (31%) was completely lost during placebo maintenance, demonstrating that the placebo effect does not last, whereas, the glucosamine effect keeps on working. The authors concluded that in spite of the fact that the treatment period was short, particularly if you consider the chronic character of osteoarthritis, a significant improvement in all clinical symptoms was evident, even after the first week of treatment.

The extent of this improvement WAS SIGNIFICANTLY LARGER WITH THE GLUCOSAMINE GROUP THAN WITH THE PLACEBO, SUGAR PILL GROUP.

Once again we see, from the chart below, a dramatically reduced overall symptoms score with the glucosamine group, yielding a far superior response. After the placebo effect had worn off, we see an increase in the symptoms with the sugar pill group. An even earlier study conducted by doctors in Mylan, Italy, in 1980, was perhaps one of the primary catalysts that instigated a rash of studies on proteoglycans, particularly glucosamines.

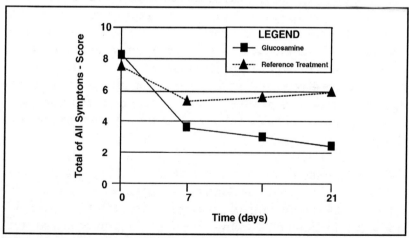

[Modified from: D'Ambrosio, E., et al., "Glucosamine Sulfate: A Controlled Clinical Investigation in Arthrosis." Pharmatherapeutica, 2(8):504+, 1981.]

Eighty patients that had severe osteoarthritis were given treatment for 30 days in a double-blind study. Participants once again were given 1.5 grams of glucosamine compared to a placebo sugar pill. Every week the researchers measured the patients' pain and joint tenderness and swelling as well as any restriction of movement. The glucosamine therapy proved exceptionally effective, yielding a 73% response rate versus a 41% for the sugar pill. It took only 20 days to reduce the symptoms by 50% in the glucosamine group and 20% of the glucosamine treated patients were completely symptom free compared to none of the 40 placebo patients. Furthermore, 29 out of the 40 glucosamine patients were considered excellent or good responders to the therapy.[7] This is exceptional and once again demonstrates the power of glucosamine. But don't forget glucosamine is an integral part of collagen type II.

Italians are not the only ethnic portion of humanity that benefits from the use of collagen derived glucosamine. A study conducted in the Philippines, once again a double-blind study, of 20 patients with osteoarthritic damage to the knee showed similar results. Within a six to eight week period the glucosamine group enjoyed significant reductions in swelling, pain, joint tenderness, at a rate of about 90% of the patients responding. Whereas, the placebo group only had about 30% of their group respond from the placebo effect.[8] No adverse reactions were reported and the level of glucosamine used was once again 1.5 grams. Thus, apparently Filipinos are able to respond to glucosamine and as we will now see, so are Thais.

A study completed at the Department of Orthopedic Surgery at Mahdol University in Bangkok, Thailand, included 60 patients, 30 receiving glucosamine injections while 30 received injections of a saline placebo. The study lasted five weeks with a four-week follow up period. Once again the results were significant, half of the glucosamine group were completely pain free, but only two in the placebo group enjoyed the same symptom relief. The overall pain score was about 90% reduced in the glucosamine group compared to about 30% for the placebo group.[9] It is obvious through double-blind, placebo-controlled studies, the best kind of studies that scientists can do, that the glucosamine moiety of collagen type II is by far the most important proteoglycan in helping to prevent, ameliorate, and repair damaged arthritic joints.

However, as important as the glucosamine is, it has an intimate relationship with the protein strands of collagen and chondroitin sulfate A, another proteoglycan that demonstrates anti-inflammatory properties. It appears that taking the entire collagen type II may be far superior to taking just glucosamine sulfate by itself. Let's now discover another important proteoglycan, chondroitin sulfate A, found within collagen type II and used to treat arthritis.

Why Chicken Sternal Collagen Type II is Superior to Glucosamine Taken By Itself

This statement is almost a contradiction because glucosamine sulfate is part of collagen type II. It is not that glucosamine is more effective than collagen type II, it can't be, because it is found within collagen type II. Collagen type II is probably more effective than glucosamine taken by itself because of the additional proteoglycans that is found therein. Chondroitin sulfates fall within this category. These wonderful proteoglycans are literally water magnets. They are composed of long chains of repeating saccharide or sugar molecules and help attract fluid to the collagen type II matrix itself. Remember that water acts as a spongy shock absorber and the water itself allows for the transfer of nutrients to the cartilage and the removal of waste. As I will show later, CSA may save you from heart disease.

In a healthy joint, the cartilage should have no blood supply. All of the nourishment and lubrication comes from the liquid that flows in and out of the joint (synovial fluid). Without this fluid cartilage becomes fragile and begins to break and crack and degenerate.

Chondroitin sulfates are the saccharide arms that jet out from a protein backbone in the collagen type II milieu. This is very much like the structure of a tree. Think of the leaves on the limbs as the proteoglycan chondroitin sulfate sections. These leaves have negative electrical charges, which repel each other, but when aligned with substances of the opposite charge they are powerful attractants. Because of their electrical charge they tend to form a stabilized web pushing each other away, but yet holding significant amounts of water. CHONDROITIN ALSO PREVENTS CARTILAGE FROM RELEASING SPECIFIC ENZYMES THAT MIGHT ATTACK AND DESTROY THE CARTILAGE AND INITIATE AN AUTOIMMUNE RESPONSE OR THE OSTEOARTHRITIC RESPONSE.

As we have seen earlier, the autoimmune response can be described as rheumatoid arthritis while the degenerative response is considered to be osteoarthritis. Chondroitin sulfates also interfere with other substances that would block the incoming nutrients getting to the cartilage. They also are involved in the production of proteoglycans, collagen type II, and cartilage matrix proteins that serve other functions. All of this is necessary for healthy cartilage to prevail. As you can see, these series of functions of chondroitin sulfates act hand in hand with glucosamines.

Chondroitin sulfate A has been studied and researched by Dr. Lester Morrison for over 30 years, in the prevention and treatment of heart attack and stroke, with profound results. See chapter 11 in this book on Chondroitin Sulfate A. This is exciting because in regard to improving cartilage function in the arthritic, we have again a naturally occurring substance derived from the collagen type II in cartilage that has no toxicity and may even help prevent the number one killer in our country, heart disease.

Chondroitin Research With Osteoarthritis Patients

In 1974, 28 patients with severe restriction of movement due to osteoarthritis were given injections of chondroitin rich cartilage extract over a three to eight week period. Of those 28 patients, 19 had excellent results, with only slight discomfort when movement was engaged in. The important consideration here is that none of these 19 people had any noticeable disability following the therapy. Six of the patients showed significant reduction in pain and could more easily move following the therapy.[10]

One of the most astounding discoveries of this study showed that the patients had relief from the osteoarthritis symptoms for seven months after the last chondroitin injection was received. This study was one of the first studies conducted by Dr. John F. Prudden with a cartilage extract in which the protein had been removed, leaving only the proteoglycans with a high concentration of chondroitin. Other studies that used chondroitin and cartilage extracts have consistently shown efficacy in terms of injection. However, as an oral supplement, studies had to be completed to determine if ingested chondroitins were as effective as the injectables.

In 1991, at the University of Naples, a six-month study included 200 patients between the ages of 52 and 75. The effects of both oral and injectable chondroitin sulfates on cartilage degeneration were observed. An interesting part of this study was that it was carefully controlled in terms of the patients' arthritic condition. In order to qualify as a patient, the patients had to have x-rays demonstrating definitive osteoarthritis as well as a typical symptom history of the disease. Other types of arthritis were excluded. The patient also had to demonstrate swelling of at least one knee joint and hypersensitivity to pressure placed on that joint, as well as pain even when the joint was resting.

The patients received either 1,200 milligrams of chondroitin sulfate orally or a 100 milligram injection of the same. The researchers concluded that all patients receiving chondroitin showed considerable improvement in their symptoms with significant loss of pain and increased mobility. No side effects were reported.[11] The oral CSA worked as well as the injectable form.

Finally, in a larger population of arthritics, a French study published in 1992, included a double blind, randomized protocol for determining the orally administered effectiveness of chondroitin sulfate compared to placebo. In this study, 120 patients with osteoarthritis of the knees and hips were given either the placebo or oral chondroitin sulfates. Additionally, all of the patients received some painkilling, nonsteroidal, anti-inflammatory drugs.

At the end of the three-month period, the patients receiving the chondroitin sulfate showed significant reduction in pain. No patients had to withdraw in the chondroitin group and an added benefit was that patients taking the chondroitin sulfate continued to experience benefits two months following the treatment period.[12] Realize that in most of these studies around 1,000 milligrams of chondroitin or more are considered to be an effective daily dose. In recalling our collagen type II analysis, approximately 14% of chicken sternal collagen type II is composed of chondroitins, therefore, taking the 3 to 6 grams daily of collagen type II yields an effective dose of chondroitins and glucosamines. Thus, simply by taking collagen type II you are giving yourself the correct dosage of glucosamine sulfate and chondroitin sulfate combined.

> *Collagen Type II Components Inhibit Cartilage Digesting Enzymes and New, Destructive Blood Vessel Formation Into the Joint*

In osteoarthritis we know that there is an initial degradation of the cartilage itself. Something is going wrong that is causing the problem. Either there is a loss of chondrocytes and proteoglycans, and a significant reduction in the renewal rate of cartilage, or there are enzymatic degradations of the surface of the cartilage occurring which allow a chewing up of the cartilage components followed by degeneration.

We know that the use of glucosamine and chondroitin sulfates resist all of these things, but researchers have recently discovered collagen type II components that are powerful cartilage digesting enzyme inhibitors and antiangiogenic (prevents new blood vessels) substances. What this means is that collagen type II literally is a powerful inhibitor of any type of degeneration of the joint at the cellular level of the cartilage itself. In a recent study, published in 1994, Drs. Koji Noyori and Hugo E. Jasin discovered specific nonaggregating collagen binding proteoglycans in collagen type II are bound to the surface of cartilage. The proteoglycans form a barrier to any kind of cell, be it a bacterial cell or inflammatory cell, adhering to intact cartilage. More importantly these specific proteoglycans resist any kind of new blood vessel formation in an inflamed joint where cartilage may be damaged.

Exactly how important these newly discovered proteoglycans are is certainly unknown at this time. Only future research will determin their therapeutic efficacy.

These particular proteoglycans are called fibromodulin (FM), fibronectin (Fn) and decorin. Thus, collagen type II itself has more proteoglycans to inhibit the early destructive process of the cartilage and prevent the formation of blood vessels that bring into the joint the inflammatory white cells that propagate the destruction of collagen type II in the cartilage. In addition to this profound effect in protecting the surface of the cartilage from initial attack from enzymes and markers from white blood cells, it may turn out that collagen type II also can protect the cartilage from these enzymes in additional ways. Researchers have recently isolated, from collagen type II, growth factors that ensure proper turnover and renewal of cartilage, protein digesting enzyme inhibitors, and collagenase inhibitors. This ensures the strength and stamina of cartilage, during normal activity and use, within the joint. How much benefit these proteoglycans are can only truely be determined by future research.

Antioxidant Promoting Proteoglycan Found Within Collagen Type II Components

Still another reason for taking collagen type II versus the individual proteoglycans such as chondroitin sulfate or glucosamine is because there is a powerful antioxidant promoting proteoglycan that has recently been identified, found within the membranes of chondrocytes. Remember chondrocytes are found within the collagen type II matrix. This substance is called cartilage matrix glycoprotein (CMGP). In order to appreciate what this particular proteoglycan means to us, it's important to review how free radicals are part of the biochemical destruction of the joint tissue in arthritis.

If we review some of the factors that can influence this disease, we know that abnormal load forces compress the cartilage and produce reduced oxygen content within the cartilage itself. When new oxygen rich synovial fluid comes back into the cartilage, it generates free radicals. Free radicals physically attack and degrade the synovial fluid component called hyaluronan and the cartilage. When pieces of the cartilage are eaten by synoviocytes (synovial cells within the joint fluid) these cells release inflammatory cytokines which prompt immune cell aggregation at the site of the joint.

The cytokines actually reprogram the chondrocytes to degenerate cartilage and with time destroy the joint. If abnormal trauma and immune cell involvement maintain free radicals, damage continues and the net result is destruction of the joint cartilage. Eating the chondro-protective collagen type II not only helps restore proper chondrocyte programming, but it also has this wonderful CMGP molecule that carries copper into the chondrocytes themselves. It may turn out that copper is one of the most chondro-protective minerals ever discovered. As we will see in later discussions on other nutritional factors that can help the arthritic, copper has proven to be very effective in helping to reduce the inflammation and pain associated with the disease. The reason is that there is a very powerful free radical scavenger within the joint called super oxide dismutase (SOD) that is dependent upon copper. The job of the CMGP, among other things, is to carry copper to the chondrocytes to ensure proper levels of the SOD. Thus we find that collagen type II carries this CMGP fraction within the chondrocyte membranes and may be another reason why eating whole collagen type II is more effective than taking the components of collagen individually.

In review, we now know that collagen type II components are truely chondro-protective agents that:

1. Resist protein cartilage digesting enzymes.
2. Reprogram destructive chondrocytes and cytokines, reducing inflammation.
3. Promote new cartilage cell synthesis, and proteoglycan synthesis.
4. Enhance the production of hyaluronan, to produce a thick, effective, lubricating, synovial fluid for the joint itself.
5. Protect the surface of the cartilage from oxidative damage and enzyme digestion.
6. Act as a powerful anti-inflammatory and pain modulator.

Thus, it is important to consider taking chicken sternal collagen type II that is more absorbable and digestible than cartilage, but yet much more complete in terms of its anti-inflammatory and chondro-protective effects than just glucosamine or chondroitin taken individually.

Dosage

Based on current research of utilizing glucosamine sulfate and chondroitin sulfate, a daily ingestion of 3 to 4 grams of collagen for people under 200 pounds is recommended, if you are over 200 pounds I recommend 4 to 6 grams daily. Always use the recommended dose first. However, if after four to six weeks of use, you have not experienced relief from pain, increase the dosage by 1 or 2 grams daily.

The components of collagen type II can produce an enormous protective pharmico-nutrient restoration of cartilage and the joint itself. This is the exciting message. This is the purpose of this book and it all began with my early research into the writing of my book entitled *Jaws For Life, The Story of Shark Cartilage* and the work of a great scientist by the name of John F. Prudden. Before we delve into the beginning of the discovery of collagen type II, it is important to note that rheumatoid arthritis is not the same disease as osteoarthritis although the end result, pain, inflammation, and destruction of the joint, is the same. Yet this destruction need not occur, for scientists have proven there is a new miracle nutrimedicine that stops this disease – Collagen type II.

CHAPTER 4

Rheumatoid Arthritis

Basically, rheumatoid arthritis, also known as rheumatism or synovitis, is a disease that is believed to begin as an infection and corresponds to those individuals who have the type of immune system that is genetically predisposed to attacking itself. Both, the infection and the genetics, work together to produce this autoimmune disease. Scientists believe that the problem arises because the infectious agents have immune stimulating properties (antigenic properties) similar to the body's own antigens and thus the immune system attacks the body as if it was a foreign invader.

Rheumatoid arthritis tends to affect joints bilaterally, both wrists, both knees, both hips, etc. Whereas, in osteoarthritis there tends to be an attack usually more severe on one side of the body. Osteoarthritis is not a disease that usually occurs after an infection, but over a period of many years in a gradual development, whereas, rheumatoid arthritis comes on suddenly. It waxes, it wanes, it comes, it goes, and it usually strikes between the ages of 25 and 50, whereas, osteoarthritis is usually after the age of 40.

In osteoarthritis usually only the joint that is afflicted is the one that demonstrates inflammation, whereas in rheumatoid arthritis we find that the inflammation, the pain, seems to be in many joints simultaneously. With rheumatoid arthritis the body reacts as if it had an infection. That is to say there is great fatigue, a feeling of sickness, fever, and weight loss, associated with this type of malady. This does not occur with osteoarthritis.

It is also interesting to know that it afflicts women past the age of 40 three times more often than men, demonstrating a probable hormone modulation. Rheumatoid arthritis may also occur in children, particularly in girls between the ages of two to five.

When doctors analyze the joint fluid they will find what is called a rheumatoid factor along with symptom identification. These combinations of symptoms and signs help to diagnose the disease. Typical symptoms include pain and inflammation of the joints, especially the knuckles and the second joint of the hand, as well as the arms, legs, and feet. General fatigue and sleeplessness along with symptomatic damage to the heart, lungs, eyes, nerves, and muscles may also occur. In the elderly it is especially important to take soothing eye drops as the corneas begin to dry and become very irritated. An excellent eye drop to use is Oxydrops distributed by Health Breakthroughs, (800) 565-7192. Muscles may also weaken, tendons shrink, and the ends of bones may become abnormally enlarged, leading to gnarled and deformed hands and feet. The pain is usually more severe upon waking up and may develop over the course of weeks or months.

If rheumatoid arthritis is treated with the new approaches of collagen type II and mucopolysaccharides associated with collagen type II, approximately 85% or more will have no permanent disability from this disease. The symptoms may endure for months or more, but after a time, especially if not treated properly, it can lead to a progressive destruction of the joint. However, if this disease is properly treated by collagen type II, the joint can be preserved, the disease can be controlled and possibly even cured.

Juvenile rheumatoid arthritis is typified by anemia and chronic fever and may also have secondary effects of heart, lungs, eyes, and nervous system involvement. In children

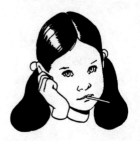

younger than five, the episodes can last for several weeks and may recur, but the symptoms are usually less severe in recurrent attacks. Juvenile cases should be treated similarly to adult cases, with special focus placed on exercise to make sure the growing joints maintain their full range of motion. Most juvenile cases can expect a full recovery with permanent damage only rarely occurring. Infectious arthritis is difficult to identify because it usually follows an injury or complication from another disease and is much more rarely diagnosed. However, many researchers now feel infection is an integral part of the rheumatoid arthritis syndrome. Bacteria, viruses, fungi, and parasites have all been demonstrated to initiate rheumatoid arthritis.

Like all diseases, no two cases are exactly alike, but all share certain symptoms. For this reason, it is important to remember the treatments may vary from case to case. Until recently there has really not been any magic bullet, as it were, that would cure all patients. Because treatment response will vary, realize the greatest response is obtained when natural therapies are combined, even though collagen type II by itself has demonstrated the most outstanding results. Remember that pharmaceuticals prescribed by a physician usually have harmful side effects. Even so, sometimes these drugs are necessary to control excruciating pain.

CHAPTER 5

Rheumatoid Arthritis and the Chicken Sternal Collagen Type II Cure

In order to fully appreciate how collagen type II has successfully been used to treat rheumatoid arthritis (RA), we must first understand the cause of rheumatoid arthritis. Basically, it is a disease that is characterized by inflammation of the lining of the joint, the synovial membranes, and an immune attack on the part of the cartilage called collagen type II, as well as destruction of the bone.

Since rheumatoid arthritis is associated with one of the white blood cell markers called lymphocyte white blood cell antigen DR4 (HLA-DR4), the disease is then known to be an autoimmune disorder meaning the body is attacking itself. Type II collagen is the substance that the lymphocyte attacks and destroys. In rheumatoid arthritis, this autoimmune component must be present in order for the disease to be manifest. Type II collagen is the most abundant structural protein in cartilage and animal research has shown, by injecting type II collagen into healthy animals, the protein induces an arthritis identical to rheumatoid arthritis in humans. When injected, the body treats collagen type II like a foreign invader and makes antibodies to destroy it. Thus, the body's white cells attack the collagen type II in the cartilage. YET, WHEN COLLAGEN TYPE II IS TAKEN ORALLY (EATEN), THE BODY TOLERATES IT LIKE A FOOD AND EVEN REDUCES INFLAMMATION TO CARTILAGINOUS COLLAGEN TYPE II FOUND IN ARTHRITIC JOINTS.

Recently, a Harvard Medical School Team reported that oral tolerance (desensitization) is an effective and nontoxic technique for suppressing the symptoms of RA. Oral tolerance is a unique and simple procedure that involves a part of the intestines called the "gut activated lymphoid tissue" (GALT). It involves feeding the patient the same substance that is being destroyed by the body's immune system. If it is the myelin sheath of nerves, the disease is called multiple sclerosis. If it is the type II collagen in cartilage, it's called rheumatoid arthritis.

Because of the GALT, a foreign protein entering the body through the digestive tract suppresses the immune response to that protein rather than increasing the immune response to destroy it. This has obvious advantages. Imagine how it would be to eat a beefsteak only to become violently allergic to beef the second time you eat it, or for that matter, any food. This is the body's way of consuming food and remaining relatively free from any kind of immune reaction to that food. A number of different research teams have studied oral tolerance in animals to suppress immune diseases resembling certain human diseases. These include multiple sclerosis, as previously mentioned, inflammation of the eye called uveitis, diabetes, as well as rheumatoid arthritis. In a clinical trial which included 30 multiple sclerosis patients, the oral administration of bovine (cow) myelin antigens decreased the number of T-cells that reacted with the myelin covering the nerves. In multiple sclerosis, the substance the immune system attacks is the myelin sheath that covers the nerves. When the nerves lose the myelin sheath, they discharge continuously and are eventually destroyed.

At Harvard University School of Medicine, Dr. David Trentham and his colleagues gave very small doses of solubilized type II collagen (from the sternums of chicks) to 10 patients with rheumatoid arthritis. These patients had all immunosuppressive drugs and anti-inflammatories such as methotrexate and mercaptopurine removed before they took the collagen type II.

Patients took small doses of collagen type II for one month and then increased the dosage for two months thereafter. The dosage was determined through the various animal studies that had determined specific concentrations. The clinical response was defined as a 50% or greater improvement in the number of swollen and tender joints, accompanied by a 50% or greater improvement in two additional measures (morning stiffness, 15 meter walking time, grip strength, Westergren erythrocyte sedimentation rate, or physician global assessment), lasting for at least two months after the treatment period. Sixty percent of the patients showed substantial clinical response and one patient showed a complete response in which the disease was totally eliminated for 26 months. More importantly, there were absolutely no side effects.

These results were so profound that a 90 day, double-blind, phase two study was conducted on 60 patients with very severe, active rheumatoid arthritis. It's important to note that these patients were not beginning or moderate cases, but the most severe cases that can usually be encountered.

Patients either received the solubilized type II collagen or a placebo. The concentration was equivalent to that in the first study. At the end of the study, 59 of the 60 patients were evaluated. Twenty-eight had received the collagen type II and 31 had received the placebo. Compared to the placebo group, the collagen type II group showed significant improvements in joint swelling, tenderness or pain. This also included the degree of swelling and tenderness together. The doctors evaluated the response in a 15 meter 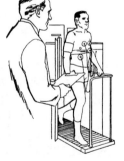 walking time at months one, two, and three. During the period at which the patients were taken off immunosuppressant drugs, those that received the collagen type II showed stability and/or even improvement while those in the placebo group tended to deteriorate. However, four of the patients in the placebo group did show a significant placebo effect. FOUR PATIENTS IN THE COLLAGEN TYPE II GROUP WENT INTO THE NEXT REALM OF THE ALMOST UNBELIEVABLE, AND SHOWED A

COMPLETE RESOLUTION OF THE DISEASE. That is correct. You have read this material correctly. These people no longer had symptoms of rheumatoid arthritis. It must be understood that no patients in the placebo group showed remission. No side effects or negative laboratory effects were seen during the study.

It is believed that by feeding type II soluble collagen to rheumatoid arthritic patients, their T-cell function is modulated either to the extent that the suppressor T-cells are triggered and migrate to the joint to block the T-cell mediated inflammation, or it just simply stops the T-cell destruction of the joint. The Harvard study was sponsored by Autoimmune a Lexington, Massachusetts biotechnology company.[13,14] Only highly purified chicken sternal collagen type II was used.

When I saw the results of this study, it was a reconfirmation of my belief that the components of cartilage hold an enormous healing potential for all of mankind, especially in regard to one of the most painful and devastating diseases we have to live with: arthritis. As I reviewed the paper and several others that described research with collagen type II, I noted two interesting aspects of the trial. First, the amount of collagen type II used was so infinitesimally small, to me it would be impossible to get any type of response unless you believed in the homeopathic principals of small dose therapy. The study actually only used one tenth of a milligram of collagen type II daily for a month, and then five tenths, one half of a milligram, for the next two months. The patients would simply pour their collagen type II powder into orange juice and drink it down. At these low dosages, it is hard to imagine the responses that were generated. However, we must realize that in rheumatoid arthritis the immune system is intimately involved, and by modulating or controlling immune response we can significantly control the attack on the joint tissues and, thus, reduce pain and inflammation. Second, four patients no longer had any sign of the disease; is this a true cure or a temporary remission? Only future research can answer this question.

Type II collagen is significant for any kind of inflammation, including osteoarthritic degeneration, and the reason is simple. The anti-inflammatory proteoglycans intertwine within the collagen matrix and this combination, in using the natural anti-inflammatory and rebuilding substances of the cartilage, literally affects immune response as well as the entire biochemistry of the joint, as we will see in a later explanation. The difference is in the dosage.

In a study conducted by T. Aigner and his associates, carefully controlled research identified the fact that type II collagen in the osteoarthritic is also degenerating as it is in rheumatoid arthritis.[15]

A more comprehensive discussion of dosage will be presented later in the book. However, it is very important that you understand that collagen type II has anti-inflammatory properties and a substance called glucosamine sulfate, which literally stimulates the cartilage producing cells called chondrocytes to produce new cartilage. At correct dosages, this can be a lifesaver for osteoarthritic patients. During my research into the studies that have been conducted with cartilage, collagen type II, and collagen fractions, I had the pleasure of speaking with several companies that were selling the chicken sternal collagen type II products. To my utter delight they had many remarkable case histories of patients that have recovered from arthritis to varying degrees. One of the first testimonials that I read addressed the problem in a very short note:

Chicken Sternal Collagen Type II Testimonials

Dear Sirs,

A short note to let you know how pleased I am with the results from using your collagen product. I am a male in my 70s, with extensive arthritis in my back and hips. I've been using collagen now for four months and thanks again.

Sincerely,
C. D. S., Boulder, CO   (testimony on file)

Another letter came to me by way of one of the companies from a woman by the name of Faith. The testimonial reads as follows:

Dear Customer Service:

While staying with my daughter and her husband over the Christmas holidays, they had two bottles of ImmuCell (containing 500 milligram capsules). Since they do not have arthritis and I do, they suggested that I take them home and see what success I would have.

I have had arthritis in my right hand for over three years and have had to have cortisone injections during that time to relieve the pain and allow joint movement. The pain would subside, but not entirely disappear. Last May my thumb was twisted back and the pain was excruciating. My doctor prescribed Relafen but it did not help. At the beginning of January, I began taking collagen type II capsules with 3 ounces of orange or grapefruit juice each morning about 20 minutes before eating. Within four weeks of taking the capsules, the pain was gone!

I still haven't received all of the strength in my hand, but it is such a relief not to have the constant pain as I've had in the past years. Also, before the Christmas holidays my right shoulder had started to become painful, and it was very difficult and painful to reach behind me or upward. After taking ImmuCell™, my movement has improved and the pain has also diminished.

I have not yet seen the complete success that I've had with my right hand, but the movement in my shoulder is comforting. I pray that as I continue the collagen type II capsules I will get the full relief I expect. Thank you for such a fine product.

Sincerely,
Faith S., California   (testimony on file)

I am a 58-year-old male who loves golf. For the past five years I played two or three times a week. Never two days in a row, as my fingers and back would hurt too much for that. In May 1996, my arthritis became very bad and I had to stop playing golf. In December 1996, I started taking MaxCTII™ collagen. After ten days my fingers stopped hurting. By February 1997, I had very little pain and not only was I playing golf, but playing two and three days in a row, carrying my bag with a full set of clubs over a 7,000 yard course.

Shelly K., in Arizona   (testimony on file)

Please, I can't urge you strong enough. If you have arthritis, and your life is nothing but pain and suffering, start taking MaxCTII™ collagen today. Stop the crippling pain and swelling and start enjoying life again!

Ray L., in Georgia   (testimony on file)

For the first time in weeks after I took MaxCTII™ collagen, I'm able to sleep without waking every two to three hours in arthritic pain.

Linda W., in Georgia   (testimony on file)

Dear Sir,

My name is John C. I am writing to you about MaxCTII™ *collagen, I saw an advertisement in the newspaper and went down and bought a bottle. My wife said, "That is a lot of money to pay for a bottle of pills that you don't know anything about." Well it was the best money I have ever spent! I am now on my third bottle and pain free from those mean arthritis symptoms! I want to thank you for making MaxCTII™ collagen. For all arthritis sufferers, it is a winner.*

Thanks again,
John C.   (testimony on file)

Gentlemen,

While on vacation in September we heard your program on the radio and decided we had nothing to lose by ordering a supply of the collagen II you were talking about. We did so and have been astounded at the results - on my Psoriasis!

I have had Psoriasis since I was 16. It started in my scalp and, over the years, simply progressed to various parts of ther est of my body. As I have gotten older it has gotten worse and, more unmangeable.

When I was 23 my body began to ache in places which had never bothered me. I was diagnosed with "tennis elbow" and given a cortisone shot. Then I was diagnosed with compressed fracture of the tailbone. I toughed it out. By 1966 the ache just didn't go away in my shoulders and back I was told I had arthritis, and was taking five aspirin four times a day in an effort to control the pain. Thus the ulcer. My doctor at that time, was interested enough to do some investigating and told me that I might have Psoriatic Arthritis.

In 1974, a trip to Merritt Hospital in San Francisco confirmed the diagnosis of Psoriatic Arthritis, they put me on 300 milligrams of Motrin. As you can see, I have lived with pain all of my adult life. I don't like it but I have learned to handle it, and the ulcer that goes with it.

There are very few publications concerning Psoriatic Arthritis, and how to cope with it. Even the Psoriasis Foundation doesn't offer much information.

My point being - I think you have touched a real winner for psoriatics. I just wish I had a few 'before' and 'after' pictures to send along. My entire back and abdomen has been covered with scales, a total of about five square feet, plus my elbows and legs with goodly portion of scaling, not to mentioned my fingernails and toenails. After starting the Colla-Cell II therapy - for the arthritis - my skin is smooth, although still red, the itching is subsiding, the scaling in my scalp in lessening, and my legs are beginning to heal. I am curious as to what the long-term effect will be on the Psoriasis.

The arthritis factor remains to be seen. It may be a bit early to be seeing any results. The Psoriatic Arthritis had 'frozen' my left wrist, there is pain and inflammation in the fingers of that hand although my fingers are still flexible. My knees and hips let me know they are still there, and now my neck is bothering me on regular basis.

My husband has felt pronounced relief in his right knee, in which the cartilage was removed when he was in the Marine Corps. He still walks with a limp but it is less noticeable. He is very pleased with the results of your product.

We have been 'spreading the word' of your product in the hope that it will be able to help others who may be facing joint replacemnt, or who, like me, have lived with pain for years.

I must add, your comment about the positive side effects have certainly been true in my case. My ulcer has bothered me very little since I have been taking the collagen II. I can now eat things that used to bother me terribly, and I am not experiencing the reflux syndrome which preiously went with the ulcer attacks.

We wish you good luck with your product. I has been a true pain-saver for us. Please keep us updated on your product and the results of its use.

Sincerely,
D. & B. R.

Dear Sirs,

I am writing to let you know how pleased I am with the results I have had with your ImmuCell Collagen Type II Chicken Sternal Cartilage 500 milligram capsules.

I have had rheumatoid arthritis for nearly twenty years. My wrists and hand are quite severly effected.

I started using ImmuCell Collagen II capsules 15 months ago in February 1997. After six to eight weeks I started to notice a big difference in pain, especially flare-ups. I have been able to reduce the mediciation I am taking. I have much less severe pain.

Thanks for putting out such a fine product.

Sincerely,
C.P. New York   (testiomony on file)

It is gratifying to know that there is a naturally occurring, nontoxic product that works even in minute doses and can have profound effects in reducing pain and inflammation.

Collagen Type II also Works on Juvenile Rheumatoid Arthritis

There is perhaps nothing more heartbreaking than to see a child crippled, with all of the promises of life taken from him or her. Certainly rheumatoid arthritis contributes its share of pain and suffering to those children afflicted with it. Now there is hope, in fact, there is an effective medicine and these children no longer have to suffer to the degree that they had before. More importantly it is my personal and professional opinion that these children will have a longer, healthier life, and even restored mobility thanks to this incredible new discovery.

In order to evaluate whether or not oral chicken type II collagen would be effective in the treatment of juvenile arthritis, Dr. Trentham and his colleagues conducted a study for 12 weeks on 10 patients with active juvenile rheumatoid arthritis. The criterion for success was the reduction in swollen and tender joints. This included a swollen and tender joint count and score, grip strength, 50 foot walking time, duration of morning stiffness, and patient and physician global scores of disease severity. Patients were assessed on a monthly basis and the results were nothing short of incredible. All the patients completed the full course of therapy. Eight of the patients (80%) had significant reductions in swollen and tender joint counts after only three months on orally administered chicken type II collagen.

The average changes from the beginning degree of swelling and tender joint counts, for the eight responders at the end of this study, were 61% and 54% respectively. The average value for other parameters showed improvement from baseline. There were no adverse side effects. The conclusion was that oral collagen type II may be a safe and effective therapy for juvenile rheumatoid arthritis, and that its use in this disease warrants additional, ongoing research.

I congratulate Dr. Trentham and his colleagues, and Dr. David Weiner, for showing the scientific world that oral tolerance can be used in the direction of arthritis. These great scientists, in my opinion, are deserving of the greatest honor that any scientific researcher can earn for the simple

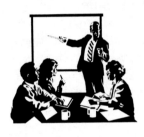

reason that they, perhaps more than any other investigators, have had the courage to use a natural product that is relatively inexpensive when compared to the pharmaceutical approach. Even without millions of dollars of funding they have been able to find a safe and effective treatment. Just think, once the world knows about collagen type II, what it means in terms of alleviating and reducing the amount of pain and suffering that people would have otherwise had to bear with this disease. Notwithstanding the temporary relief given to patients with painkillers and anti-inflammatories, as well as nonsteroidal anti-inflammatories, we must always realize that these medications have side effects. They can and should be used when they are needed, but not on a long-term basis.[16]

The future of collagen type II as an oral treatment for rheumatoid and osteoarthritis is very bright, and it may turn out that collagen type II can be effective in preventing the rheumatoid arthritis form of this disease from ever expressing itself. In 1995, English scientists tolerized mice with type II collagen. This tolerance procedure rendered the animals resistant to the induction of collagen type II arthritis. The authors of this study proposed that the self-tolerance procedure could have great potential in the application to preventing human rheumatoid arthritis.[17]

It may even turn out that the use of oral collagen type II on a daily basis can prevent forms of joint inflammation other than rheumatoid arthritis. Dr. Weiner's group studied the effect of orally administered type II collagen in antigen-induced arthritis (AIA). Lewis rats were given oral doses of collagen type II before these animals were given arthritis by injections of bovine serum albumin. Also, Freund's complete adjuvant, a substance commonly used to induce the arthritic condition, was used. Joint swelling was significantly reduced using minute dosages of collagen type II. These researchers concluded that oral collagen type II could suppress arthritis in an animal model in which immunity to collagen type II did not play a role. In other words, it was not rheumatoid arthritis. It appears that collagen type II may prevent the two most common forms of arthritis.

Interestingly enough in this case, the effect was dose dependent and immunity occurred at the lower doses. This research clears the path for future investigations to determine if oral collagen type II, if taken on a routine basis, could reduce or prevent human inflammatory joint disease from various causes. The reason that collagen type II would probably work as a preventive measure is because even in traumatized joints where there is no overt history of rheumatoid arthritis, we can find degeneration of collagen type II and a subsequent antibody production.[18] At this point it is important to understand how the immune system interacts in order to appreciate the mechanism by which oral collagen type II can be of assistance to not only the rheumatoid arthritic patient, but also the person suffering with osteoarthritis. Later, in my discussion on joint disease, I will also discuss many other diseases that afflict the joint that may have a beneficial response to oral collagen type II.

CHAPTER 6

A High-Tech Explanation of Nature's High-Tech Defense System and the Collagen Type II Connection

We hear a lot about the immune system, but what precisely is immunity? When we come into this world we are met with an assault of many different agents that can harm us. This endless supply of harmful agents can trigger a response by our immune system, which is the mechanism established to protect us.

This is known as biological immunity and is the most powerful disease fighting weapon in the world. Its basic job is to distinguish friend from foe. That is to say, to identify and destroy a virus rather than identifying and attacking our joint cartilage. Among the many infectious agents, the greatest threat and the most elusive enemy to medical science is the virus. Today we face an onslaught of infections from new strains of bacteria and viruses as well as the common cold virus.

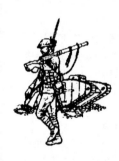

Let's consider our body's defense system as an army. First, we have immune cells that originate in the bone marrow and mature in the lymph nodes, spleen and gut associated lymphoid tissue (GALT). These anatomical laboratories produce the white blood (soldier) cells called leukocytes. The thymus gland is an important player in this battle. It produces hormones that help these leukocytes reach maturity and become aggressive to fight the enemies.

Lymphocytes are special leukocytes and are known as T-cells. The T-cell soldiers separate and acquire specialized mobilization functions. Each is called by names that reflect what they do in the process of defending our bodies. Some become 'killer' cells which attack microbes or cancer cells directly. Others become 'helper' or 'suppressor' cells.

Another important leukocyte born in the bone marrow matures in the GALT and is known as the B-lymphocyte. These B-cells are the cells that produce antibodies. Bone marrow also produces scavenger cells that go in between the cells to kill and clean up dead viruses, bacteria or chemicals that don't belong there, and they are called phagocytes.

There are other cells that act as 'mediators'. These cells, along with biochemicals, play vital roles in our defensive army. Acting together, they create a deployment strategy that would cause MacArthur, Patton, and Attila the Hun to stand back in awe.

The body's lymphatic and circulatory systems carry these immune substances through the body to where infection has made an in road. The immune army marches to areas where the blood vessels are so narrow that defending soldiers must pass through in single file. Not only does the circulatory system carry these important soldiers to defend the body from the enemy, it also carries them to the mammary glands where all of the major components of our immune system are concentrated in the first milk. Some of these specialized cells produce what are known as immunoglobulins and cytokines. The immunoglobulins, primarily IgG, IgM, IgA, and secretory IgA, are used by white blood cells (leukocytes) to manufacture the necessary antibodies. Cytokines are the immuno-regulatory chemicals that either speed up or slow down the aggressiveness of the immune system in terms of its attack on a particular enemy.

In regard to cytokines, there is a division of these chemicals into various immune modulators. They include about a dozen interleukins, of which interleukin-4 and 10 are extremely important to rheumatoid arthritic victims. Other arthritis inflammatory *modulators* are tumor necrosis factor (TNF) and several interferons.

Nature has used the oral route for the development of the immune system since the origin of mammalian species. There is little doubt that the immune system, immature at birth and depressed at aging, needs to be boosted and kept alert by assisting the body's production of cytokines. When an infant is given mother's milk (the first milk, colostrum), there is an enormous number of cytokines, immunoglobulins, and growth factors that assist in awakening and activating the baby's own system.

It is a known fact and proven in scientific studies that breastfed infants have fewer colds and other infections. They also have fewer autoimmune diseases later in life. And this, then, is one of the key features about keeping our immune system vigilant against the enemy, yet passive against it's own body's tissues.

T-lymphocytes secrete the cytokines that bind to target cells, and mobilize many other cells and immune substances. They encourage the growth of cells, they trigger cell activity, direct cell traffic, destroy target cells, and arouse the cleanup crew known as phagocytes. Let's now apply this understanding of our immune system to the induction of a rheumatoid type of arthritis and see how collagen type II is so critical in recovering from this disorder.

In both osteo- and rheumatoid arthritis there is a collagen type II breakdown in the initial part of the disease, and this breakdown can be increased from the production of cartilage destroying enzymes. The primary structure of cartilage consists of collagen type II that is intertwined with the proteoglycans and noncollagenacious matrix proteins and water.

Collagen type II by far is the most prevalent and important protein of the cartilage. Collagen type II resists tensile forces and serves as an organizing skeleton that helps to maintain the structural integrity of the cartilage. Fourteen different types of collagen have been identified. Cartilage specific collagens are type II (principle component), type IX, type X, and type XI. The type IX collagen is believed to be the actual 'glue' that holds the other type II latticework of articular cartilage together.

Degradation of type IX collagen by proteolytic enzymes has also been identified in the primary stages of both osteo- and rheumatoid arthritis. This degeneration leads to an 'ungluing' of the collagen type II scaffold and has been proposed as the mechanism for degenerative changes in both types of arthritis.[19]

Inflammation in the joint is also influenced by a series of substances, which the body derives from fats, called eicosanoids. Eicosanoids can, in turn, produce proinflammatory prostaglandins or anti-inflammatory prostaglandins. The joint destruction in arthritis is also modulated or determined in some part by the amount of free radicals. These are the metabolic terrorists that arise from the release of hydrogen peroxide from white blood cells and the destruction of super oxide dismutase, one of the most important anti-inflammatory, free-radical scavengers in the joint chamber.

Scientists have now determined that the cytokines that increase inflammation are tumor necrosis factor (TNF) interleukin-1 and interleukin-6, as well as colony stimulating factor-1 (CSF1). These are secreted primarily by activated macrophages, the clean up crew. However, the lymphocytes also secrete interleukin-2 (IL-2), interleukin-3 (IL-3), interleukin-4 (IL-4), and interferon gamma (IFN-gamma), some of which reduce inflammation.[20]

Activated macrophages keyed into destroying the type II collagen in the cartilage and lymphocytes can also produce eicosanoids and free radicals, which have very powerful inflammatory actions. Thus, the two primary inflammatory and anti-inflammatory modulating chemicals are eicosanoids and lymphokines. They can also determine the degree of cell proliferation, the amount of collagen digesting enzyme produced, known as collagenase, and other collagen digesting enzymes called proteases.

They also have the capacity to induce bone reabsorption and can actually produce collagen vascular diseases. However, to counterbalance these modulators, as in all of nature's biochemistry we find balance, transforming growth factor-beta (TGF-beta) is produced by the synovial fluid and platelets. This can suppress T-helper cells, natural killer cell proliferation and activation, and even block free-radical generation.

Synovial fluid, platelets, and lymphocytes can also inhibit (cartilage digesting) collagenase production, which benefits the rheumatoid arthritic patient. Essential fatty acids derived from fish oils, cold-pressed flax seed oil, and other natural healthy sources provide the precursors for the anti-inflammatory prostaglandins, the good eicosanoids. They also suppress T-cell proliferation, IL-1, IL-2, and TNF production. This has long term benefit for both rheumatoid arthritic and lupus patients.

Even a form of vitamin D_3 has been shown to block inflammatory lymphokine and TNF production.[21] Thus, dietary manipulations can have powerful benefits for arthritic victims.

What Animal Research Tells Us

Interestingly enough, the very method by which doctors induce rheumatoid arthritis in animals, utilizes that part of the cartilage which first breaks down in both rheumatoid and osteoarthritis, soluble collagen type II. Chicken sternal collagen type II induces an autoimmune arthritis when injected into susceptible strains of mice. In fact, researchers have actually identified the very part of the collagen that induces the rheumatoid arthritis type of disease. It's called the cyanogen bromide fragment (CBII) of collagen type II. The way that scientists determined that the CBII was the culprit was to take CBII and immunize laboratory animals before the injection of collagen type II to induce rheumatoid arthritis. If the animals were immunized prior to the injection with CBII, they simply never acquired the disease. Therefore, researchers are now determining that this particular peptide, CBII, is the fraction of collagen type II that is the primary tolerogen that can significantly alter the course of the disease.

The question is, "What starts the destruction of collagen type II initially to allow the CBII to be exposed and generate an autoimmune response?" Most investigators now believe that an infectious agent must be the primary inducer of this destruction. This can be a bacteria such as that which causes Lyme disease, it can be a virus such as a relative of the parvo virus that causes a fatal infection in dogs, it can also be a parasite such as the *Nigleria amoeba* parasite.

This implies that early control of infection can help prevent this disease from expressing itself. For right now, we must understand that arthritis can be induced in laboratory animals by the injection of native collagen type II. The progression of this experimental autoimmune disease can be induced in primates as well as rodents. It is used widely, as a model of the disease process, for experimenting with potential therapies. The immunology of collagen type II induced arthritis has compelling parallels with human disease, and was the basis on which the oral tolerance collagen therapy was actually developed.

Using the animal model called 'collagen-induced arthritis' (CIA). Researchers have determined that the T-helper cells, the lymphocytes that actually help in the production of antibodies, and the other lymphocytes that participate in the progression of rheumatoid arthritis have what are called surface markers. Researchers have blocked these surface markers to prove that they are intimately involved in the disease. If by blocking them the disease no longer progresses, then these markers become a crucial and pivotal feature in the progression of the disease. Lymphocyte markers so far determined in the literature are CD_4, $CD_{40}L$, and MHC class 2. Thus, we now know that the disease progression is dependent on the T-cell, particularly the T-helper cell (CD_4). If laboratory animals are given an anti-CD_4 treatment before the collagen type II induced arthritis is administered, then there is relatively no rheumatoid arthritis that develops.[22]

It has also been established in the literature that suppressor lymphocytes (CD_8), the ones that suppress the production of antibodies toward collagen type II among other things, if increased can very much suppress the disease. Consequently, there is acceleration with CD_4 and a braking CD_8 system that allows for a control of immune response to the collagen. However, it has been thoroughly established that rheumatoid arthritis suppression by the administration of oral collagen type II is an active suppression of the T-helper cells and the B-cells (antibody producing cells), probably through the regulatory action of interleukin-4, interleukin-10, and TGF-beta.[23]

The mechanism by which oral tolerance seems to work is that the oral collagen type II is consumed and travels down the intestines and, finally, is absorbed by the gut activated lymphoid tissue (GALT). The collagen is absorbed with the activation of the T-suppressor cells (CD_8+T) which triggers a specific and nonspecific suppression of the antibody production at the level of the joint cartilage through the cytokines already mentioned.

One of the more fascinating discoveries about the oral tolerance effectiveness of collagen type II is when researchers induced rheumatoid arthritis not using collagen type II injections. When other antigens such as mineral oil were used, they discovered that if the animals were pretreated with collagen type II these inducers of the disease were not effective. What this in essence means is that regardless of what is destroying the collagen type II within the cartilage, collagen type II will probably be very effective as an oral tolerance suppressor of the disease. The simple reason is that be it a bacteria, virus, parasite, or trauma, it seems to be a protein digesting enzyme reaction that leads to the release of collagen type II destruction of the joint. By giving collagen type II prophylactically, research is showing that it is a very powerful inhibitor of rheumatoid and other forms of arthritis.[24]

The use of oral type II collagen may also be shown in future research to be useful against other types of diseases in which type II collagen destruction is involved. In fact, specific collagen typing for these different diseases may also be a key feature. For instance, the current debate over whether or not silicone in breast implants can induce autoimmune disease.

Breast Implants and Collagen Type II

It is interesting to note that the manufacturers of breast implants, as well as the official spokespersons for the Medical Association, claim that there is no significant data to indicate that breast implants are increasing autoimmune disease.

However, research is beginning to focus in on the fact that silicone, a foreign synthetic chemical, can negatively impact the immune system so as to provide the basis for an autoimmune reaction. Researchers have determined that silicone gel breast implants increase the frequency of auto antibodies to collagen types I and II.

In one study, 70 women without any specific autoimmune disease, using the very criteria of the American College of Rheumatology to show an autoimmune disease, were given silicone breast implants and were studied for the presence of serum antibodies to human type I and II collagen. Another group, this time consisting of 82 women, with systemic lupus erythematosus (SLE), and 94 women with rheumatoid arthritis (RA), as well as 133 healthy controls were also studied. There was a higher frequency of autoantibodies to collagen in each of the groups when compared to healthy controls. This simply meant that silicone induced autoantibodies to collagen with or without symptoms being expressed.

From this research and other data, it is clear that silicone can induce reactivity to collagens by enhancing the immunogenicity process.[25]

In an earlier study, these same researchers determined that the breast implant silicone induced a stronger antibody reaction to type I collagen, whereas women with lupus and rheumatoid arthritis reacted more toward the type II collagen. The women with lupus reacted more weakly to both. The reactivity of women with silicone implants suggests that silicone or its biodegration products can act as adjuvants to enhance immunogenicity toward collagen.

When my wife was 28-years-old, she suffered with fibrocystic disease, and had to have both breasts removed. She was one of the first to receive the newly formed silicone gel implants. Over a period of years, she did not have any abnormal immune problems, however, beginning in her forties, she began to have some difficulties, which included more frequent infections and visual problems. Because of the lawsuit that was popularized on the mass media between DOW Chemical and many women who had claimed their failing health was due to silicone, my wife and I decided to see a physician.

Upon examination, he determined that the breast implants had solidified and scar tissue had formed with probable leaking of the silicone. Upon having the silicone breast

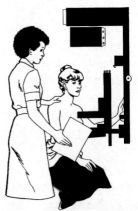

implants removed, one breast implant burst and spilled silicone throughout the breast cavity. Almost immediately following the surgery, my wife began to complain of unusual health problems. Her eyes would flicker and she began to lose feeling in her fingers and her toes. She had severe lapses of memory, and was sleeping from 10 to 15 hours daily. I then decided to take her to one of the top neurologists in the country, and after $4,000 of sophisticated diagnostic tests, the neurologist claimed that she had the beginning of what is known as multiple sclerosis, an autoimmune disease. I immediately took her to a homeopathic clinic in Nevada that had saved my health 14 years prior, and they made her a vaccine type of medication called a *homeopathic nosode*. Within a period of two months, all of the symptoms had dissipated.

Interestingly enough, one of the nutritional therapies that I initiated for her was shark cartilage at a level of about 3 grams daily. Shark cartilage contains, as other cartilages do, collagen type II. Chicken sternal collagen type II was not available at the time. Over the past seven or eight years, my wife's health has remained fairly good and occasionally she will have relapses. However, once the vaccine nosode is renewed, the condition abates. Currently she is taking collagen type II as well as a series of antioxidant vitamins and essential fatty acids. For more information about this clinic, call (800) 552-8885.

In one of the more significant animal studies, researchers actually took silicone gel from commercial breast implants and injected them into Dark Agouty rats. Within a short time, the rats developed arthritis.[26]

> ## Orally Administered Collagen Type II Blocks Arthritis Caused by Breast Implant Silicone

Dr. S. Yoshino has previously shown that silicone injected into the joints of rats could induce arthritis. He has also tested the new hypothesis of oral tolerance with collagen type II. Rats were fed collagen type II either before or after intra articular-injection (articular joint cartilage) of silicon. Dr. Yoshino and his group found that feeding collagen type II EITHER BEFORE OR AFTER THE INJECTION OF SILICONE MARKEDLY SUPPRESSED THE DEVELOPMENT OF CHRONIC ARTHRITIS.

The oral antigen did not affect the early phase of acute joint inflammation, but there were no proliferative responses to collagen type II of lymph node cells from rats that had the silicone injection. The proliferation of collagen type II of lymph node cells from collagen type II primed rats was markedly suppressed by the addition of spleen cells from animals fed collagen type II. Furthermore, these results indicate that the T-cell mediated arthritis is down regulated by oral administration of collagen type II and that this, in turn, dramatically reduces joint inflammation and helps prevent the lymphocytes from further destroying collagen type II in the joint cartilage.[27]

Armed with this new dramatic information, it would seem to me that every woman in this country that has a silicone breast implant should be using collagen type II. We know that the breast implants, whether they are ruptured or not, will leach silicone into the tissues. Silicone is a foreign synthetic chemical and has the capacity, as has been proven in animal research, to induce autoimmune diseases including arthritis.

For the first time we may now have one of the most powerful methods and products for protecting women from silicone breast implant autoimmune disease. In 1997, my wife began taking collagen type II and continued her nosode injections, and she remains symptom free.

With the animal studies indicating that oral collagen type II can produce a tolerization to the autoimmune response caused by the breast implant silicone material, it would be logical for every woman who has the breast implants with silicone to be on collagen type II. Furthermore, because lupus patients as well have demonstrated antibodies to collagen type II, it would also be an important adjuvant therapy to be used with these patients. Other seemingly unrelated diseases, such as Menier's disease and myopia, may have a "collagen" connection.

CHAPTER 8

Menier's Disease, Myopia, and The Collagen Type II Connection

Another disease that may respond to oral collagen type II tolerization is Menier's disease. This is basically a disturbance of the labyrinth in the inner ear. It is seen with a great variety of conditions such as drug poisoning, atherosclerosis, even infectious disease such as syphilis and blood dyscrasias. Inflammation of the eighth cranial nerve and tumors of the brain can produce Menier's symptoms.

The patient often has a severe ringing in the ears with a sudden onset, also deafness, nausea, vomiting, and dizziness, which may last for several days to several months. The treatment varies depending on what is causing the disease, symptomatic treatment involves the use of sedatives and withholding fluids due to the tremendous edema of the labyrinth of the ear. In severe unresolved cases, a special operation severing the affected branch of the auditory nerve seems to help.

There may be a strong connection in Menier's disease with the formation of antibodies to collagen type II. In a recent study, Menier's patients were tested along with 22 normal volunteers serving as controls and matched against 28 rheumatoid arthritis patients, and nine patients complaining of dizziness. Serum antitype II collagen antibodies were measured in all groups. The purpose of the study was to determine if there was a possible connection with the autoimmune destruction of collagen. The immune response in Menier's disease was quite dramatic. Menier's patients exhibited high serum antibody levels to type II collagen compared to controls. The highest levels were found, however, in rheumatoid arthritis victims. This means that there could be an immune response to type II collagen within the ear in Menier's patients. The results suggest the development of certain immune abnormalities that lend support to the idea that an immunological disorder plays a key role in some cases of Menier's disease. If this is true, oral tolerization with type II collagen may prove to be significant therapy for these Menier's patients.[28]

Other researchers have found high antibody levels to type V collagen in Menier's disease as well as type II.

Myopia and Collagen Type II

Oral collagen type II might be very helpful for progressive myopia. One of my colleagues, who is world renowned for his clinic specializing in the alternative healing of cancer, has had progressive myopia since his youth. It is very disheartening to see a person gradually lose his vision with this, supposedly, genetically inherited disease.

As an eye doctor I frequently saw high near-sighted people, but the progressive form of myopia is not that common. One of the problems with progressive myopia is that it can be induced and aggravated by extensive reading.

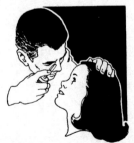 Researchers have determined that over the years as a person reads, the downward slope of the eyes along with the muscles converging the eyes tend to raise the intraocular pressure. As this pressure is exerted on the globe of the eye, if the connective tissue of the eye is unstable or weak, the axial length of the eye will actually increase, putting the focal point in front of the retina. This is known as near-sightedness. As years pass and the eye continues to enlarge due to this pressure, there is a progressive thinning of the retina with subsequent tears, detachment of the vitreous (the jelly in the back of the eye) and ultimate loss of vision and blindness can occur.

In a study measuring the antibodies for collagen, researchers took the blood serum of 55 patients and the lacrimal fluid of 23 others. Serum antibodies to collagen were detected in 50 to 70% of the patients with all forms of myopia (congenital, early acquired, and acquired at school age). Antibodies to the collagen were not detected in the tear fluid, which was regarded as evidence of the fact that the connective tissue disorder was that of a systemic (blood) autoimmune type. Antibody titers were highest in the blood serum of patients with uncomplicated and slowly progressing myopia. Interestingly enough, the rapid, progressive type of myopia complicated by the various ultimate degenerations of the parts of the eye including the vitreous, as well as ruptures of the retina, was characterized by a deficit of antibodies to the collagen in the blood serum.

This implies a possible protective role of antibodies to collagen detected in the blood of patients with myopia. These results are regarded as a proof in favor of autoimmune reactions to collagen in the development of medium and high myopia. It is my hope that researchers will now take the next step and start using type II collagen on various types of myopia to determine a possible therapeutic benefit. Imagine not having to get thicker and thicker contacts and glasses and, more importantly, preserving your retina and vision in later years. Collagen type II may not only be our connection with good health, but also with good vision.

CHAPTER 9

Correct Dosage for Oral Tolerance and How It Can Save You the Pain of Arthritis

Oral Tolerance is a mechanism that allows the immune system to become less aggressive toward itself. It is in that sense of the word that a true modulation system is kind of like the brake on an automobile. You don't want the car to go too fast and a braking system is definitely required. Low doses of an orally administered collagen type II protein which is the actual structure that is destroyed in arthritis, if taken orally, suppresses the production of the white blood cells that are literally attacking the cartilage. It also reduces, therefore, the production of inflammatory cytokines that provide for the inflammation, which in turn reduces pain. Collagen type II increases the anti-inflammatory cytokines, IL-4, IL-10, and TGF beta that suppress the other cytokines that cause the inflammation.

However, there is an additional mechanism by which the orally consumed antigen works. It goes to the gut-associated lymphoid tissue and has an influence on the T-helper cells, which has the effect of reducing the attack on the collagen in a nonspecific way. Scientists call this *bystander suppression.* Thus, it may not be necessary in some cases to identify the specific target autoantigen, in the case of arthritis it's the collagen type II, in order to suppress an organ specific autoimmune disease by oral tolerance. It is necessary only to administer an orally effective protein capable of inducing regulatory cells that secrete suppressive cytokines.

In the case of rheumatoid arthritis, this is precisely what happens and this is why collagen type II is probably going to be very effective on osteoarthritis as well. If it is going to subdue those inflammatory cytokines by increasing the anti-inflammatory cytokines, it is going to work on any kind of inflammation of the joint. There are a large number of studies that have shown that the primary mechanism by which this works is called active suppression.

Another mechanism by which the oral tolerance can be working has recently been described as clonal anergy. This is defined as a state of T-Lymphocyte unresponsiveness due to absence of proliferation. Thus, as the T-Lymphocyte proliferation decreases, the inflammatory cytokine production diminishes in proportion.

Note the chart on the following page and see that there are literally two ways of inducing tolerization, one is with low dose ingestion of the autoimmune protein collagen type II and the other is high dose ingestion. In high doses of orally administered antigen the antigen passes through the gut and enters the systemic circulation either as intact protein or antigen fragment. This creates a condition in which the helper cells, the cells that help stimulate the production of antibodies and inflammatory cytokines, are set into a state of unresponsiveness and anergy. Start with (low dose) 2 or 3 grams daily for four to six weeks and then increase your dosage to 4 to 6 grams (high dose) to improve joint function.

Dosage

The amount of collagen type II to be consumed to inhibit the progression of rheumatoid arthritis or even osteoarthritis is dependent on several factors. In the original research conducted on oral tolerization using collagen type II, minute doses (from 1 to 5 milligrams daily) were utilized. These dosages are so minute that it would be difficult to administer this level of collagen type II on a consistent basis. Furthermore, the collagen used would have to be extremely purified and standardized so as to represent a

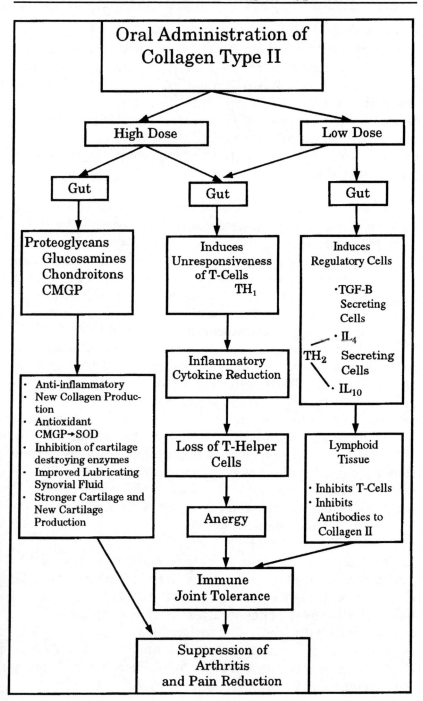

pharmacological product versus a health food store product. It may turn out that the collagen type II with the associated mucopolysaccharides (proteoglycans such as glucosamine sulfate and chondroitin sulfate A) would be far more attractive due to the fact that the higher doses could diminish both osteo- and rheumatoid arthritis as well as other inflammatory diseases. The overall goal is to REDUCE PAIN and that is precisely what the dosage is intended to do.

In support of the theory that collagen type II can reduce inflammation, pain, and destruction of the arthritic joint, an animal study was published in 1993. Researchers took laboratory animals and induced arthritis with a substance called pristane. If the animals were pretreated with type II collagen, it lowered the incidence of the pristane-induced arthritis in direct proportion to the amount of collagen type II consumed. In other words, increasing doses of orally administrated collagen type II lowered the incidence and severity of the pristane induced arthritis.[29] Thus, because of the research indicating higher dosages can be more effective, the collagen type II association with the proteoglycans may turn out to be more significant when 3 to 6 or more grams daily of the product are consumed. The "type" of arthritis you have is important also. If you have rheumatoid arthritis, always start with a low dose first (3 grams). Then, increase it after four to six weeks of use. If you have osteoarthritis, you may start with higher doses, 4, 5, or even 6 grams daily.

Regardless of what dose you start with, use only highly purified chicken sternal cartilage derived collagen type II. Chicks, six to eight-weeks-old, have collagen type II that holds the highest concentration of glucosamine sulfate, chondroitin sulfate A and other proteoglycans. The companies I recommend carry this high quality product. Realize that as the word gets out on collagen type II, many other companies will carry a quality product.

Analysis of Collagen Type II
(derived from chicken sternal cartilage)

Calories per 100 grams	375
Calories from fat	0.9
Solids Protein (NX5.55)	66.6%
Carbohydrate (by difference)	26.34%

The proteoglycans glucosamine and chondroitin sulfate A contain both protein and carbohydrate (sugars). A careful analysis of collagen type II derived from chicken sternal cartilage found:

Glucosamine to be 14.3% of the solids
Chondroitin Sulfate A to be 14.2% of the solids.

Fat		0.1%
	Total Solids	94.37%

Ash, %		8.28
Sodium	mg/100 grams	774
Potassium	mg/100 grams	1961
Calcium	mg/100 grams	530
Magnesium	mg/100 grams	–
Zinc	mg/100 grams	–
Iron	mg/100 grams	1

Aino Acid Profile (grams / 100 grams product)

Arginine	4.42
Histidine	2.05
Isoleucine	2.90
Leucine	4.20
Lysine	3.54
Methionine	1.38
Phenylalanine	2.14

Analysis of Collagen Type II
(derived from chicken sternal cartilage) cont.

Threonine	2.60
Tryptophane	0.37
Essential Amino Acids	
Alanine	4.51
Aspartic Acid	5.29
Cystine	0.46
Glutamic	8.75
Glycine	8.93
Hydroxyproline	3.90
Proline	5.25
Serine	2.45
Tyrosine	1.16
Valine	2.43

CHAPTER 10

Collagen Type II is More Than You Think

The Anti-inflammatory Proteoglycans of Chicken Sternal Collagen Type II

If we take a look at healthy cartilage, we find that the primary protein is collagen, composed of about 5 different kinds of collagen, the primary one being collagen type II. Intertwined, interwoven, and intermixed with the collagen type II strands are the proteoglycans: chondroitin sulfate A and glucosamine sulfate. These mucopolysaccharides form a web, a web that holds water. This dense web has collagen type II and proteoglycans so tightly and densely bound that the cartilage becomes one of the strongest and one of the most powerful connective tissues we have.

One of the primary purposes of the chondroitin sulfate A and glucosamine sulfate are to help hold water in the dense meshwork of cartilage. The proteoglycans are an essential element of healthy cartilage, for besides holding water, they lubricate and nourish the cartilage itself. If cartilage becomes damaged either from trauma or cartilage digesting enzymes from bacteria, the netting becomes weak, detached, loses its tensile strength, stretches out of shape, and in the process the essential proteoglycans are lost. Without these waterholding substances, the cartilage loses its ability to absorb shock, it begins to degenerate, it forms cracks, and begins to erode. Eventually the cartilage is completely worn away and now allows bone rubbing on bone with tremendous friction and destruction.

Of the several mucopolysaccharides found intertwined within the collagen type II, we see that glucosamine sulfate stimulates specific cells, that actually produce the cartilage components, called chondrocytes. An interesting feedback system exists within the cartilage milieu. If the glucosamine is found in abundance within the collagen type II, it ensures the chondrocytes will produce more of the proteoglycans needed to form the waterholding matrix. However, if glucosamine is reduced, fewer proteoglycans are made. The water will be lost. The integrity of the collagen type II and the cartilage are then compromised. Remember healthy cartilage and healthy collagen type II are dependent on the level of glucosamine found therein. Also remember, six-week-old chicken sternal collagen type II has the highest level of glucosamine.

For the arthritic suffering the excruciating pain of this disease, glucosamine goes to the final step. Studies have clearly shown that it can reduce pain dramatically and improve joint function in those suffering with arthritis. The studies have been conducted primarily on osteoarthritis.

The most common form of glucosamine is glucosamine sulfate. Glucosamine also makes up 50% of hyaluronic acid, which forms the backbone of the proteoglycans such as chondroitin sulfate A. Thus, glucosamine occupies the pivotal position within the collagen type II itself in terms of connective tissue synthesis. The building blocks of collagen type II are amino acids, especially proline, glycine, and lysine. However, the building blocks for proteoglycans are sugars. Collagen is so plentiful it makes up one third of our total body protein content and is our most common protein. The other major components are the proteoglycans. Thus, cartilage reflects, in a rather interesting and accurate way, the body's composition of connective tissue. Proteoglycans are large molecules, and when they complex together to form long chains of modified sugars, the correct term is glycosaminoglycans (GAGs). It is interesting to note that glucosamine is made from a precursor molecule that is essential for energy itself called glucose, blood sugar. The conversion of glucose to glucosamine by the chondrocytes is, in fact, the rate-limiting step for the production of proteoglycans.

For all arthritis sufferers, here is the good news. Orally ingested collagen is well absorbed and finds its way to the collagen type II and ultimately into the form of proteoglycans. Eating solubilized collagen type II will give you sufficient glucosamine to do the same.[30] Research has shown over 70% of glucosamine sulfate is absorbed and within 24 hours it finds its way to the synovial fluid of the joint as well as the cartilage.

Do Infections Cause Rheumatoid Arthritis?

Joint inflammation has been shown to develop soon after or during an infection that has occurred elsewhere in the body. This type of arthritis is known as reactive arthritis. How is it that an infection at a distant part of the body can create an inflammation in the joint tissue when it seems that it is so unrelated? The answer to this question is not completely understood, but we do know this; some forms of microbes, especially bacteria, have a foreign protein material called an antigen that resembles the same protein materials in other tissues such as our joints. When the immune system cues in to destroy that particular protein in the bacteria, it automatically does the same to the protein in the joint. Fortunately, only a small percentage of our population has this type of reaction, which means that the susceptibility of an autoimmune response known as rheumatoid arthritis is genetically predetermined.

In the case of those who acquire rheumatoid arthritis, the individual must have a particular kind of T-cell receptor to a specific antigen peptide found by a self-major, histocompatibility complex molecule (MHC). Specific transport molecules in our blood stream carry bacterial or foreign microbial antigens to the T-cells (specific white blood cells). This then alerts the T-cell to destroy that particular antigen. In the case of rheumatoid arthritis, there is a strong association with the HLA-B27 antigen that is carried by some bacteria. Thus, T-cells recognize the foreign antigen when the HLA molecule of the immune system presents them. In some people, especially those who have the HLA-B27 type, antibodies are produced to this antigen. A molecular mimicry provokes the T-cells to attack the joints that contain the self-antigens. Thus, even though a bacterial infection may occur at a different part of the body, the white blood cells wind up in the joint attacking the tissues that biochemically look like the bacteria.

This structural mimicry of the bacteria antigens causing a harmful cross-reaction to healthy body tissues can include the following rheumatic diseases:

Rheumatic Fever
Rheumatic fever is caused by a species of streptococcus bacteria and, if allowed to progress without antibiotic treatment, can cause secondary conditions in which there is a swelling of the brain, spinal cord, joints, and damage to the kidneys and heart.

Chlamydia-Induced Reactive Arthritis
Chlamydia trachomatis is now recognized as the most prevalent venereal disease in the western world. A more common name that is attributed to this type of reactive arthritis is called Reiter's Syndrome, and is secondary to the sexually transmitted infection. There is a great deal of evidence that the trachomatous infection is found in up to 61% of the cases of Reiter's syndrome. Successful treatment of the disease with long acting antibiotic therapy has been effective in stopping the inflammation and pain associated with the infection and should be the treatment of choice with this disease.

Gonococcal Arthritis
In addition to the Chlamydia-induced arthritis, another venereal disease, gonorrhea infection is also capable of producing a reactive type of arthritis. Prompt recognition and treatment of this common disease results in a cure and elimination of the problem.

Syphilitic Arthritis

Syphilis is not a disease of the past. It is a disease of the present, and most probably the future. It has become a very significant clinical problem and in spite of the fact we have more powerful types of antibiotics today, syphilis can cause a secondary arthritis with a wide variety of symptoms including arthritic pain. Once again, the disease is effectively controlled if detected early and treated with antibiotics.

Lyme Disease

Lyme disease is a multi-system, tick-born disorder caused by the spirochete bacteria known as *Borrelia burgdorferia*. The disease symptoms begin as a skin rash, but quickly manifest joint pains and inflammation. The nervous system can also be involved with various forms of paralysis or partial paralysis. Laboratory diagnosis is important and blood antibodies are measured against the infected organism. Along with the other diseases, antibiotic therapy is the normal therapy of choice. However, there are a number of natural products, the most powerful of which is the colloidal silver. In fact, I have seen several cases of Lyme disease resolve completely with the use of colloidal silver, the most important of which was the case history of Dr. Paul Farber, a chiropractor, nutritionist, and naturopath.

Dr. Farber was literally paralyzed with Lyme infection. He rediscovered the over 60 years of medical use of colloidal silver that, actually, was the key factor in his recovery. I have interviewed Dr. Farber on numerous radio shows and he has a plethora of recoveries of patients, with many different kinds of infections, with the application of colloidal silver. Because the rheumatoid version of arthritis is initiated most likely by infectious organisms, and as we shall see later, can be anything from bacteria to virus, it is my opinion that colloidal silver should be employed as a standard part of the therapy along with the collagen type II. Use the collagen type II simultaneously while using antibiotics or colloidal silver.

Candida Arthritis

Interestingly enough, *Candida albicans* can induce a form of reactive arthritis. Because this disease is a fungus, it is very difficult to treat and has many dietary inducers (sugar foods). Once again I encourage those who have chronic yeast infection to reach for colloidal silver. No known organism can resist silver. Silver is the most powerful, natural, antiviral, antibacterial, and antifungal agent. It is interesting to note that *Candida albicans* is not the only fungus that can create arthritis. There are several other species of fungi that have been shown to cause musculoskeletal infection. Again, use collagen type II at the same time you are trying to control the yeast infestation.

Parvovirus, B$_{19}$ Infection

Not only do dogs get parvovirus, but also a particular species of parvovirus known as B$_{19}$ has been recently discovered and characterized as a DNA virus that affects humans. Interestingly enough this discovery of the B$_{19}$ infection shows that it is common and widespread among human populations. A number of clinical syndromes have been ascribed to this infection. The B$_{19}$ virus causes adult skin rashes and rheumatoid-like polyarthralgia (pain in the joint). Once again, colloidal silver will be our most powerful protector from this virus. Modern medicine has few effective antiviral products. Almost every one of them causes serious side effects if taken over an extended period of time. For this reason colloidal silver, because it's lack of toxicity, can be extremely effective in helping to stave off the B$_{19}$ infection. Don't forget collagen type II as part of your treatment.

HIV - AIDS

Although controversial, researchers have demonstrated that HIV infected patients do manifest rheumatological symptoms. I'm going to refer to my book *AIDS, Ozone, and the Nutritional Stimulation of the Immune System* that discusses life saving strategies using natural and low toxicity pharmaceuticals. To order this book call toll-free (800) 565-7192.

Human Leukemia Virus Infection
Retro viruses can cause rheumatic disorders and the human leukemia virus is no exception. The lubricating joint fluid has been shown to contain, in rheumatoid disorders, the HTLV-1 organism.

Parasites
Parasitic infection can also induce a variety of rheumatic disorders if these organisms infect specific tissues. This can include muscle tissue, connective tissue, tendons, as well as the joint itself. Perhaps the most popular proponent of the parasite theory of rheumatoid arthritis is Dr. Roger Wyburn-Mason. This investigator has taken the joints of deceased rheumatoid arthritis victims and placed the synovial membranes (lining of the joint) in a bath of water, with warm water on one side and cold water on the other. His technique was designed to stimulate any parasitic organisms to invade the warm water from the joint tissue and avoid the cold. This is precisely what happened when he experimented with these joints. In six out of every ten rheumatoid arthritic victims, he was able to recover the *Nigleria amoebae* parasite, which basically is a one-cell creature that, he feels does tremendous damage to the joint tissue. The elimination of this organism through the use of antiparasitic drugs and medication promotes recovery. Use collagen type II simultaneously with the antiparasitic drugs in order to speed up recovery.

Dr. Mason went on to show that by giving the drug, Flagyl, he was literally able to cure six to eight out of every 10 rheumatoid arthritic patients. As an eye doctor, I had a patient that was the husband of a singer on the Lawrence Welk show who, unfortunately, had suffered from severe rheumatoid arthritis. This man's pain and crippling arthritis was so severe that his wife had to drag him on a beach towel to the bathroom in order for him to relieve himself. After having exhausted every form of therapy, this gentleman sought the services of Dr. Mason. Having taken his treatment for a period of six months, he was walking normally once again. The only difficult problem I had was giving this man an eye examination as he was bragging about his success and would not stop.

It is my recommendation that colloidal silver be used as it may turn out to be as effective as the standardized forms of antiparasitic drugs. In cases of rheumatoid arthritis and these rheumatoid diseases where an infection or parasitic organism plays a role, there is a side effect that can occur called the "Herxheimer Reaction." This is basically a die off reaction of the infectious organisms. As they die they release poisons into the blood stream that cause a severe fever and inflammation. This is not a pleasant situation and the patient should always be under the care of a physician when this type of therapy is employed. Just another reason to use collagen type II during treatment.

It is interesting to note that herbalists for years have claimed the powerful, natural antibiotic herbs such as Taheebo and garlic, as well as blackhorn have been successful with arthritic victims.

Other Microorganisms Associated with Arthritis

Besides the microorganisms already discussed, several other bacteria that infect the intestines can cause reactive arthritis. These include Yersiniae, Salmonellae, Shigillae, and Campylobacters. Campylobacters has been renamed *Helicobacter pylori* and has recently been shown to be the primary causative agent of ulcers. Salmonellae is a common food poison and Shigllae, as well as Yersiniae, have been shown to infect the intestines as well.

Staphylococcus aureus is one of the most common bacteria in this world, it seems to be everywhere and heretofore has not been associated with rheumatoid arthritis. However, researchers have isolated *Staphylococcus aureus* strains from patients with septic arthritis and found that the bacteria possess a collagen receptor, which apparently provoked the rheumatoid type of disease. Apparently, the collagen receptor is both necessary and 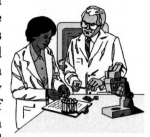 sufficient to mediate bacterial adherence to cartilage in a way that allows the bacteria to damage the cartilage releasing collagen type II and setting up the autoimmune response. Laboratory animal experiments with *Staphylococcus* have shown that this is capable of inducing the rheumatoid type of collagen type II induced arthritis. Another microbe that can be involved in augmenting the arthritic condition is a virus known as the Cytomegalovirus (CMV). CMV infection has recently been shown to damage blood vessels and possibly be a contributing factor to atherosclerosis. CMV by itself can cause a serious disease in humans, however, researchers have taken rat CMV and found that it actually augments collagen type II induced arthritis with increases in immune reactivity toward type II collagen.

Summary

Reactive arthritis has been demonstrated to be associated with infection. As I have shown, it can be parasitic, bacterial, fungal, or viral. It is often associated with inflammation of the urethra (urinary tube), conjunctivitis (inflammation of the lining of the eye), and sometimes skin rashes. It characteristically follows an infection usually of the gastrointestinal or genitourinary tract and in this particular kind of arthritis, antibiotics are extremely helpful. However, because of the resistant forms of staph and strep and some of these other organisms, colloidal silver may be one of our greatest benefactors in terms of a therapy for this type of arthrosis. Don't forget to take collagen type II to reduce inflammation and the immune response to joint collagen.

Spondyloarthropathies

Ankylosing spondylitis is a form of rheumatic disease that is characterized by inflammation of the spine, hips, and joints other than the knees. Just as the disease of rheumatoid arthritis that afflicts the knees is associated with a genetic marker HLA-B27, so is the ankylosing spondylitis. There is a strong association with the HLA-B27 marker with at least six different subtypes of this disease. Just as rheumatoid arthritis has a cross reactivity with an infectious organism so does the ankylosing spondylitis. The chart on the following page summarizes this rheumatoid affliction that is immune mediated.

Note the diagram on the following page showing that the first response is the T-Lymphocyte which responds to the bacterial infection. The bacteria peptide is attached to the HLA-B27 marker. This marker then stimulates production of antibodies and these antibodies in turn will attack the joint cartilage tissue whether the cartilage tissue is in the knee joint, in one of the articulating facets in the spine, or in the hips. Wherever the cartilage is found, the antibodies will be attacking it and creating pain and inflammation. This is the so-called autoimmune reaction of rheumatoid disorders.

Other Therapies You Can Use With Chicken Sternal Collagen Type II
➤ Eat whole foods, including fruits, vegetables, grains, nuts, cold water fish, and other sources of essential fatty acids.

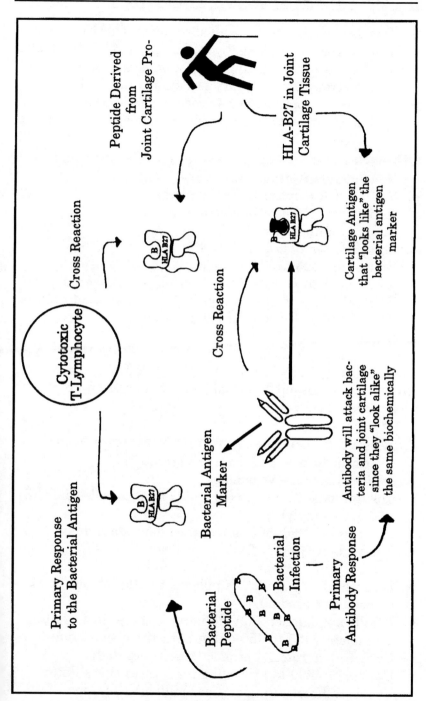

➤ Exercise, particularly the affected joint. This can be done through yoga, stretching, hydrotherapy, and other exercise that will use the full range of motion of the joint, without adding strain that will further damage the joint.

➤ Use dietary supplements, as needed, to relieve the pain and inflammation, and to help repair the damage already done.

Other Suggested Supplements for Osteoarthritis

◆ Niacinamide: 1 gram, three times daily.
◆ Vitamin B Complex: Daily supplement.
◆ Antioxidant Group: Daily supplement
◆ Boron: 3 milligrams, three times daily.
◆ *Boswellia serrata*: 4 grams daily.
◆ Bromelain: 125 to 450 milligrams, three times daily.
◆ Essential Fatty Acids: Fish oil such as salmon oil or cod liver oil. If you prefer vegetable oils, try cold-pressed flaxseed oil or Evening of Primrose oil.

Note: After using chicken sternal collagen type II, you may not need any other supplements. Even so, a multiple vitamin, mineral and essential fatty acids can improve your general health.

Suggested Supplements for Rheumatoid Arthritis

• Check for food sensitivities or malnutrition.
• Avoid nightshade vegetables.
• Collagen type II: 6 to 12 (500 milligram) capsules daily (3 to 6 grams daily)
• Pantothenic Acid: 500 milligrams, four times daily.
• Antioxidant Group: Daily supplement.
• Boron: 3 milligrams, three times daily.
• Essential Fatty Acids: Supplement with fish oils or cold-pressed flax seed oil.
• DL-Phenylalanine: 750 milligrams, three times daily.
• Bromelain: 125 to 450 milligrams, three times daily.
• *Boswellia serrata*: 4 grams, three times daily.
• Curcumin: 400 to 600 milligrams, three times daily.
• Colloidal Silver: (50 parts per million) 1 teaspoon daily.

CHAPTER 11

Chondroitin Sulfate A (CSA) Saves Joints, Hearts, and Blood Vessels

Chondroitin Sulfate A Benefits	
✦ Antitumorogenic	✦ Improves Rheumatoid
✦ Antiatherosclerotic	Arthritis
✦ Antithrombotic	✦ Increases RNA and DNA
✦ Improves:	Synthesis
Liver Diseases	✦ Fights Migraine
Nerve Disorders	Headaches
Heart Function	✦ Fights Peptic Ulcers
✦ Lowers Cholesterol	
✦ Increases Bone Strength	
✦ Improves Osteoarthritis	

Chondroitin Sulfate A (CSA), found in collagen type II, is not a drug, but a nutrient that acts like a drug, without the harmful side effects. Although it is not as potent as a blood thinning prescription pharmaceutical, such as heparin, it exerts some profound effects on circulation and has proven extremely beneficial in reducing the risk of death and/or further deterioration from cardiovascular disease. In biochemical terms, it is, as mentioned earlier, a proteoglycan (mucopolysaccharide) and is in the same family as substances such as the glucosamines, hyaluronic acid, and dermatin sulphate.

This mucopolysaccharide is an essential part of the cartilage that lines the ends of bones, and is extracted for use as a human dietary supplement from shark, ray, and other higher vertebrate skeletons, such as the ends of cattle and pig bones, and the tracheal rings of cattle. However, the highest concentration of CSA is found in chicken sternal collagen type

II. It is also found in the exoskeletons of insects and crustaceans, red and brown algae, and the cell walls of bacteria and fungi. CSA is a major constituent of cartilaginous and collagen tissue from the intervertebral disks, tendons, sternum, nasal septa, aorta, and the cornea of the eye. Also present to some extent in all organ systems, CSA can even be extracted from the brain,[31] so it is certainly not unnatural and already very much a part of the body. As a main component of collagen type II, it is extremely useful for treating a variety of ailments, especially circulatory problems.

Long before it was ever used in any clinical procedures, chondroitin sulphate A was recognized in the form of protein complexes. In 1861, two investigators first isolated and identified chondroitic acid.[32] In the same year, Rudolph Virchow proposed that a deficiency of the constituents of cell walls, specifically the mucopolysaccharides, was part of the cause of arteriosclerosis (hardening of the arteries).[33] In 1889, CSA was discovered by C.T. Morner when he isolated a crude extract of chondroitin-4-sulfate which he called chondromucoid.[34] Elie Metchnikoff, a Nobel prize winner, discovered in 1909, that the cells of connective tissue, such as cartilage, helped alleviate infection and inflammation.[35] The work of these pioneers, although done with crude extracts, forms the foundation of much of the modern research.

Another pioneer in the field of CSA research was Dr. Karl Meyer of Columbia University. In the 1940s, he coined the term mucopolysaccharides, a formal designation for the entire family of complex sugar proteins, also referred to as proteoglycans or glycosaminoglycans.[36] A wealth of information has been published on this subject, especially in the past three decades, most of it coming from university medical centers.

There are myriads of applications for CSA in a clinical setting; so many, in fact, that there would not be space for all of them in one volume. L.A. Crandall discovered as far back as 1936, that CSA was useful for the treatment of migraine and idiopathic headaches. Its benefits as an antitumorogenic agent have been researched lately,[37] and in Germany much has been done to explore the substantial benefits of injecting CSA for the treatment of osteoarthritis.

Oral use has also proven effective for the treatment of structural load-bearing disorders, including arthritis. Taking collagen type II with its CSA may provide a problem-solving alternative to costly joint-replacement operations. Also of note, is the work of the Italians using CSA as a treatment for peptic ulcer. In the United States, Dr. John Prudden, of the Columbia University College of Physicians and Surgeons, has found that CSA is a potent anti-inflammatory agent.[38] In addition to these, other therapeutic applications include use for liver disease, nervous system conditions, and even some psychosomatic complaints.[39]

The focus of my discussion, in this chapter, will be on the use of CSA in the improvement of cardiovascular problems. Most of us are aware of the dangers of arteriosclerosis, or disease of the circulatory system. This condition is dangerous because the arteries are literally what carry life-giving blood to the entire body; without the circulatory system, our cells, tissues, and organs would have no way to get nourishment and energy, expel waste, or fight off disease. This life sustaining system is not merely a bunch of tubes interconnected like some fantastic intracorporeal subway system, but a delicate network requiring proper maintenance and care in order to function properly.

The arterial walls are comprised of collagen, elastin, enzymes, mineral complexes, mucopolysaccharides, and other organic substances. These molecules interconnect in a delicate balance to form the arterial wall, but are subject to damage and deterioration brought on by excess fat, oxidized cholesterol, smoking, pollution, diet, stress, and genetic factors. Because one of the main components, collagen type II, contains a great deal of CSA, we can see why using collagen type II as a dietary supplement might help restore cardiovascular health.

The effect of CSA on cardiovascular health can be seen most profoundly in the aorta, the largest blood vessel leading from the heart. In the aorta, CSA is responsible for water retention, viscosity, permeability, and maintaining a proper molecular balance in the arterial wall. It stabilizes the elastic fibers that act as a barrier against the infiltration of oxidized fat molecules, which cause the formation of lesions on the arterial wall.

Unfortunately, as we grow older the levels of CSA in the arteries and bloodstream drop. This can lead to serious trouble for the health of arterial walls. The fat, cholesterol, and free radicals in the bloodstream are always present, but in varying levels depending on the diet. The damage they can cause to the cell walls is like a fire burning next to a wood building. As long as the fire fighters can keep enough water on the building and on the fire, it will stay in control and not do any damage. But if the water pressure lowers, the fire will start to get out of control. The fire is like free radicals. First, it will dry out the building, then actually burn holes in the walls, and The clogging of the arteries occurs when the inner lining, made mostly of elastic tissue, breaks down and cholesterol and other fatty materials collect in the lesions caused by free radical damage. This inner lining contains a great deal of CSA. So when CSA levels are low, the lining, or arterial intima, is more likely to be damaged. Young individuals who still have relatively high levels of CSA are able to protect themselves against this damage, but as we get older and CSA levels get lower, the level of protection goes down.

This damage can be circumvented by the use of oral supplements that contain CSA. Many researchers today feel that oral CSA supplements can help to prevent the buildup of plaque on arterial walls due to atherosclerosis, as well as arthritis and other degenerative diseases associated with aging. One of the best things about collagen type II CSA supplementation is that it is not a wonder drug that may have unknown side effects, but is part of the body's natural defense against degeneration, and is already found in the circulating blood.[40] Supplementing this is merely returning the body's CSA to its previous levels, making it one of the active ingredients in the fountain of youth, called collagen type II.

One of the most significant characteristics of CSA is its antithrombogenic or anticoagulant effects, since these factors play a major part in the prevention of heart attacks. Basically, thromboses are blood clots that may clog the walls of arteries that have been narrowed by the buildup of atherosclerotic plaque. When this clogging occurs, blood flow to the heart is stopped, resulting in a heart attack, if it occurs in the brain it can cause a stroke. While clotting is an important natural process that prevents us from bleeding to death in the case of an injury, if the blood clots too easily, which can happen as CSA levels get lower, a thrombosis may form. In addition, a high fat diet and other factors associated with aging can also cause the blood to clot more easily. In individuals who do not get sufficient exercise, these blood clots can form in the major arteries of the legs, become dislodged, and travel through the bloodstream to the heart or brain where the damage is always severe and many times fatal.

Although many physicians prescribe anticoagulants to prevent this from occurring, collagen type II CSA supplementation is a natural means of reducing the risk of blood clots. Extensive studies, which I will discuss next, have been performed detailing the use of CSA for patients with coronary heart disease. While most of the early studies were performed with rats, monkeys, and other animals, human subjects have been used in the most recent studies, and have shown very promising results. A significant finding of these studies is that patients suffering from angina had a significantly lower incidence of thrombosis or blood clots when taking CSA supplements, and angina pain was less intense, of a shorter duration, and often subsided completely.

The benefits of CSA continue outside of the reduction of thrombosis. First, it also aides in regulating cholesterol. Dr. K. Murata, of the University of Tokyo, conducted tissue cell cultures investigating the effects of mucopolysaccharides on cholesterol. When exposed to small amounts, cholesterol levels were reduced more so by CSA than by any other of the other proteoglycans tested. Additionally, CSA possesses anti-inflammatory, antiallergic, and antistress properties. It strengthens bones both after fractures and in postmenopausal osteoporosis, as well as increases synthesis of RNA and DNA at the cellular level.[41]

Dosages of CSA can be taken orally, such as collagen type II, or through injection, or topically. Topical applications quicken the growth of new bone tissue after experimental bone defects are created. Patients with arthritis, osteoarthritis, and other inflammatory diseases of connective tissue have found similar success using a cream rich in CSA.

Not only is the use of CSA an effective measure in the treatment of these diseases, but it is also extremely safe. When using any nutrient or drug, it is important to be aware of the side effects, if any, associated therewith. Over the 40 years that CSA has been used for the treatment of these medical conditions, no cases of toxicity have been reported in the medical literature. The only potential side effect is an allergic reaction, but these are usually due to impurities resulting from the extraction process rather than an actual allergy to CSA. (For this reason it is extremely important to obtain a product in its natural form such as collagen type II).

Even in Japan, where CSA is used by more than 20,000 people every day, no cases of toxicity have been reported over the 40 year history of its use. Dosage levels as high as 10 grams daily have been used for periods as long as six years, and no signs of toxicity have been observed. This indicates that there are no chronic, long-term side effects of using CSA. The lack of side effects and the substantial benefits make CSA a great medical breakthrough; it is a potent, natural, nutritional supplement without the potential dangers of a synthetic drug.[42]

Not only does CSA supplementation eliminate the side effects of synthetic pharmaceuticals, but it also helps to maintain the natural, youthful balance of mucopolysaccharides found in young, healthy bodies. It is ridiculous, of course, to think that we can live forever simply by taking certain supplements. But by using antioxidants, like vitamins C, E, and A, and using other supplements, such as collagen type II with CSA, to protect our cells from free radical and environmental damage, it is reasonable to hope that degenerative diseases may be prevented, and the extra years we are afforded will be happy, healthful, and prosperous.

This hope of better health has been the quest of adventurers for hundreds, even thousands of years. The search for a fountain of youth led people around the world, but now it leads people to spend years doing research to find a better cure for the diseases that cause us to feel old and broken down. Such is the case with Lester M. Morrison, M.D. This great scientist has spent decades doing research on the benefits of taking CSA for the treatment of cardiovascular disease, and his research will be the focus of this next section. It is amazing to see how, over the years, the positive effects of CSA supplements not only continued, but also even improved. These results are remarkable, considering that pharmaceutical treatment usually starts off with a strong positive effect, but eventually tapers off as a tolerance develops and higher doses are required to achieve even minimal benefits.

My discussion of Dr. Morrison's research will cover his findings from studies he published beginning in 1968, and detailing his work with a group of 120 patients with coronary artery disease. The patients were divided into two groups, 60 receiving CSA therapy, and 60 serving as controls. As we will see, the 60 patients receiving the CSA fared much better than the controls, and provided evidence to substantiate the claims made about the benefits of CSA for the treatment of coronary artery disease, as well as other types of dysfunction of the circulatory system.

CSA is present in normal circulating human blood at a concentration of 1.5 milligrams per liter.[43] In organ tissue culture studies conducted by Dr. Morrison and coworkers, it was found to be the most effective of several therapeutic agents for reducing the lipid content in the blood of humans, other mammals, and birds. This "clearing" effect was shown in various organs, including aorta and arterial tissue. CSA has also shown some growth stimulating properties in tissue and organ cultures, leading to an increased production of DNA and RNA.[44]

Other researchers have found that a single application of CSA effectively reduced lipids and lipoproteins from cells of the human coronary artery, aorta, and other arteries in tissue cultures prepared within four hours postmortem.[45] Interestingly, the younger the subject, the faster the clearing of the cells.

This information led to further investigations to determine the therapeutic effectiveness of CSA when administered orally to a series of patients with clinical coronary artery disease or coronary arteriosclerosis. This research is especially pertinent, considering that cardiovascular disease and its complications are the leading cause of death in the United States today.

To test the effectiveness of CSA, animal studies were first conducted where it was found that CSA reduced the incidence and severity of atherosclerotic lesions in squirrel monkeys, rabbits, and rats fed an atherosclerotic diet.[46,47] IT ALSO PROMOTED THE LIBERATION OF CHOLESTEROL DEPOSITS FROM ARTERIAL WALLS IN HUMAN SPECIMENS, which is likely a reason for its success in preventing cardiovascular incidents in the human subjects.[48-51]

The difference between the treatment group and the controls in the human studies was plainly evident after only two years of treatment. The control group experienced 15 cardiovascular incidents in the first two years, compared with only one in the treatment group (keep in mind that all of the subjects had coronary arteriosclerotic disease, making all members of both groups prime candidates for heart attack or other cardiovascular problems). The 15 incidents in the control group consisted of eight heart attacks, four of which were fatal, and seven cases of coronary insufficiency, indicating an impending heart attack. The CSA treated group experienced only one cardiac incident, that being a fatal heart attack. As mentioned earlier, the CSA was well tolerated by all the subjects receiving it, with no signs of toxicity.[52]

The reasons for the effectiveness of CSA treatment on these human subjects are more apparent when animal studies are evaluated. In a study of squirrel monkeys, atherosclerosis was artificially induced in order to study the effects of CSA treatment. The squirrel monkey was selected because this subhuman primate is different from many animals in that it can develop atherosclerotic lesions in the aorta and coronary arteries that are similar to those of an adult human male. Also like humans, these monkeys rarely develop these lesions when young, but as they age, the frequency and severity of atherosclerotic lesions increases. The location, development, and severity of atherosclerotic lesions in these squirrel monkeys makes them ideal subjects for use in testing the development and treatment of atherosclerosis in human beings.[53,54]

In this experiment, eight squirrel monkeys were obtained from a compound in Colombia at approximately two and a half to three years of age. They were fed a diet of monkey chow and fresh fruit for five years, during which time they maintained a good state of health and had minimal changes in body weight. After five years they were divided into two groups, both relatively equal with respect to sex and size of the subjects. The first group was the control group, to whom a daily injection of sterile saline solution was administered. To the second group an injection of saline solution with 20 milligrams of CSA was given. The diets remained the same for both groups.

After 90 days of this treatment, the animals were sacrificed and frozen sections of the basal portion of the heart were prepared for examination. Ten sections were randomly selected from each animal and examined without the researcher knowing to which group the section belonged. Each section was graded on a scale of zero to four with zero indicating no lesions and four indicating severe lesions.

In the control group, three of the four monkeys had lesions averaging two in severity, with one of the control females being without such lesions. Of the CSA treated monkeys, none of them had atherosclerotic lesions. The medial part of the apex of the heart was also sectioned. It was found that the monkeys receiving CSA treatment had significantly fewer signs of the development of atherosclerosis than did the control group. The controlled environment of this experiment helps substantiate the possibility that CSA can not only prevent, but reverse the effects of atherosclerosis in squirrel monkeys. Similar findings have resulted from studies conducted with rats and rabbits. Because of the similarity in the development of atherosclerosis in humans and squirrel monkeys, it is likely that the effects of CSA are the same; similar prevention and regression of the disease is probable in humans taking CSA as a supplement to their diet.[55]

Dr. Morrison and his coworkers have conducted studies on the way in which CSA and other acid mucopolysaccharides function in the body. Their findings indicate the following in relation to the development of atherosclerosis. In tissue and organ cultures CSA stimulates cellular growth, and RNA and

DNA synthesis. It cleared from aorta and coronary walls the lipids, lipoproteins and cholesterol plaque that were building up on the cell walls. Electron microscope studies with C14 cholesterol indicate that CSA increases turnover of fats and fatty acids within the cells, act as a metabolic regulator in a hormone-like manner. Studies with rats indicate that CSA is effective in the prevention of coronary atherosclerosis, and that it accelerated the regression of atherosclerosis, but not of coronary artery calcium deposits or fibrosis. Interestingly, only orally administered CSA resulted in the prevention of coronary atherosclerosis.

Chondroitin sulfates and other acid mucopolysaccharides were found to be effective anticoagulants when administered by injection. Even when rats were fed cholesterol and toxic doses of vitamin D in order to induce the adhesion of cholesterol and other lipids to the arterial walls, those animals that were given CSA did not have plaque buildup in the arteries. In angina patients given CSA at a dosage of 10 grams daily for 90 days, thrombus formation time (the stickiness of blood cells) was greatly increased in comparison with controls. When administered over periods of six weeks to 12 months, chondroitin sulfate A and chondroitin sulfate C lowered serum lipid and cholesterol levels 20%. All of the chondroitins A, B and C are bound to collagen type II.

These effects may be due to the defensive actions of the mucopolysaccharides. CSA and similar substances act as part of the body's natural defense system, and are among the first cells to respond to the damage of arterial walls by any foreign substance. Any time damage is done to the arterial walls by any foreign substance, the primary function of many of the mucopolysaccharides is to repair, regenerate, and grow normal new tissue.[56]

Armed with this information, it is not surprising that after three years, the 60 human subjects receiving CSA were doing much better than the control group. In three years the CSA group had only four coronary incidents, including three fatal heart attacks, and one coronary insufficiency. The control group had 29 coronary incidents, comprising of six fatal heart attacks, 10 nonfatal heart attacks, eight cases of acute coronary insufficiency, including one recurrent case, and five cases of myocardial ischemia (reduction of blood flow to the heart).[57]

Studies done on rats indicate that the effect of CSA is one of regeneration of arterial tissue as well as elimination of fats and cholesterol from the blood. This is based on Dr. Morrison's finding that rats fed a diet designed to cause atherosclerosis led to the development of severe damage to the heart and surrounding arteries, but only one sixth of the rats given the same diet plus CSA experienced such damage. The two groups had the same levels of fats and cholesterol in the blood and liver, but the CSA apparently led to the healing of any damage that otherwise would have been done by these substances. Think of it as an 83% improvement in arterial protection.

In a similar study, rats that were given a nonatherogenic diet (a diet that would not induce atherosclerosis) and rats given an atherogenic diet plus CSA were found to have a higher number of life saving branch arteries from the heart than were rats given an atherogenic diet, but no CSA. This further indicates the effectiveness of CSA in the prevention and reversal of damage done to the cardiovascular system by fat and cholesterol.[58]

CSA that has been used by Dr. Morrison and his associates for these studies was shown to have a molecular weight of 29,500, which may be important for achieving optimum results. When the molecular weight is reduced 3,000 to 8,000, the antiatherogenic and antithrombosis qualities are either absent or greatly reduced despite the increase in absorption from the gastrointestinal tract. It is also important to get CSA in its natural state such as that found within collagen type II. When it is extracted from bovine trachea or nasal septa by gentle means, it has different properties than when extracted from whale or bovine skeletons by harsh methods of extraction. Apparently while both are technically pure CSA, one may have antiatherogenic effects, while the other has cholesterol-lowering effects. For this reason it is important that CSA be obtained from collagen type II in its natural state in order to achieve the desired therapeutic or preventive effects. If CSA is degraded through the extraction process it may not be useful for the prevention of thrombosis and atherosclerosis, which are the actual dangers of high blood lipid and cholesterol levels.

The reduction in danger is statistically apparent in the study of Dr. Morrison's 120 test subjects. After four years, the control group had 36 coronary incidents, while the CSA treatment group had only six.

Every year in the USA there are 500,000 deaths from acute coronary incidents, and an equal number of surviving cases of acute coronary thrombosis or heart attacks. If these were added to the equal number of incidents of acute coronary incidents, there would be a total of some two million coronary incidents annually. It is conceivable that the effectiveness of CSA would be the same for this broad group as for the 120 patients in the study group, meaning that CSA could lead to the elimination of well over one million cardiac incidents every year.[59]

The long-term use of CSA continued to benefit the 60 test patients. It is rather unfortunate that there has to be a control group in an experiment such as this one, since the control group had 38 coronary incidents, nine of which were fatal. Contrarily, the CSA group had only six coronary incidents in five years, four of which were fatal. The control group had nine fatal and 10 nonfatal heart attacks, one fatal and 12 nonfatal acute coronary insufficiencies, and six acute myocardial ischemias. In comparison the CSA group had four fatal heart attacks, and two acute coronary insufficiencies. Even after five years, there were still no laboratory abnormalities or signs of toxicity in the CSA group. The treatment was well tolerated by all the patients.[60]

After six years of treatment with chondroitin sulfate A, the death ratio compared to controls was 4:14. Furthermore, the ratio for the occurrence of coronary incidents was 6:42. Statistically there was found to be a 99.9% probability that the differences between the treatment and control groups was due to the treatment with CSA, further indicating that it is this variable that led to the success of the treatment group. Also of note is that all 120 patients that took part in this study continued on their traditional treatment regimen (if they were on one when the treatment began). This means that the incidents in both groups occurred despite the fact that they were receiving treatment for their condition from a regular physician. This treatment would have included pharmaceutical and dietary measures.

The study involving the 60 CSA patients certainly showed that chondroitin sulfate is a potent supplement for the prevention of coronary incidents, and in the animal studies helped to prevent or reverse the disease. For the sake of finding the most effective supplement available, Dr. Morrison and coworkers conducted a study in which different types of cartilage and mucopolysaccharides were evaluated for their effectiveness in a treatment regimen. According to the first experiment, in which animal sources were compared to pure chondroitin-4-sulfate, these sources were nearly as effective as commercially extracted pure chondroitin-4-sulfate. This simply means collagen type II would have the same effect, if not better, since the CSA is in the highest concentration in the collagen type II fraction of the cartilage. Collagen type II is more easily digested than cartilage. The second experiment also included plant sources and found that Irish moss was a good source, with thrombus (blood clot) formation times nearly equal to those in the commercial and animal samples. Mucopolysaccharides extracted from rice bran were actually found to have some coagulant activity, indicating that extracts from this source should be avoided. This study indicates that there are several biologically potent sources of CSA mucopolysaccharides that can be used for the replacement of arterial cells damaged by atherosclerosis, but the best is chicken sternal collagen type II. Although these are not the only sources available, according to the research they are the most effective in reducing blood clotting, atherosclerotic buildup, and the life-threatening coronary incidents.

While all of these statistics certainly provide convincing evidence of the benefits of taking CSA as a dietary supplement, I would like to share with you some remarkable recoveries from my own experience. It seems that we can read statistics about animal studies or groups of people, and remember them long enough to learn the name of the supplement, and think about getting some for ourselves or a loved one that is suffering. When we learn about how a natural therapy has helped an individual, someone, perhaps a mother, brother, friend, or dear associate, it becomes imperative that the problem be dealt with. For this reason I would like to tell of the progress that I have seen using natural therapies to treat circulatory dysfunction.

In 1986, I was part of a research team put together to test a vitamin mineral CSA supplement designed to treat circulatory diseases developed by Dr. Yiwen Tang, M.D. Dr. Tang was born and raised in Peking, China, did his undergraduate studies in Lyon, France, and then moved to the United States where he studied at Harvard University to become a physician. This international experience opened his mind to the vast array of treatments available for different diseases, unlike many western physicians who simply prescribe whatever the big pharmaceutical companies are promoting at the time. He studied traditional Eastern and Western medicine, and was knowledgeable about the different treatment possibilities that were currently available. As we will see in the following examples, his experience has proven valuable with the effectiveness of a CSA rich product designed for the treatment of circulatory problems.

The first patient in the study was a 47-year-old lady that we will call Mrs. B.R. Mrs. B.R. had diabetes and had undergone heart bypass surgery before going to Dr. Tang's clinic in Reno, NV for treatment. Tests were made to evaluate the amount of circulation through her blood vessels before treatment and then again after three months. She was facing having her feet amputated due to poor circulation. The CSA-rich product led to improvements in the hardness of her arteries and speed of blood flow after only 90 days. Circulation returned to her feet and she no longer had to have her feet amputated. Furthermore, she said that she felt much better and had five of eight pulses, that were reduced before treatment, begin to return to normal. This is definite clinical evidence of improvement. Five years after she had taken the CSA rich product she attended one of my lectures and wore sandals to show everyone she still had her feet.

Mr. W.N., a 71-year-old man, had high blood pressure, high cholesterol, and generalized hardening of the arteries (arteriosclerosis). A radionuclide angiogram taken before treatment began, measuring physiologic pump function, muscle and valve function, and heart wall motion, was abnormal. This test provides similar information as a coronary angiogram, or arteriogram, but without placing a catheter inside the heart, and with a much lower level of radiation exposure. This is done with the use of a multilens, high-speed camera, and is ideally suited for noninvasive study of outpatient treatments, such as the CSA product. After only three months of treatment, Mr. W.N. showed significant improvement in eight of nine measurements taken with the radionuclide angiogram.

CSA seems to have played a definite role in the improvement of these patients, and provides further evidence for the usefulness of noninvasive methods for treating circulatory dysfunction. The results presented here would certainly justify further scientific investigation into the possibility of nutritional and orally administered treatments for mild to moderate cases of circulatory dysfunction.[61]

Medical science has led us to some amazing breakthroughs in high-tech treatments for diseases. Because cardiovascular disease is the number one killer in the United States today, it seems that much of the research and development has been focused in that area. Although things like artificial hearts, balloon angioplasty, valve replacement, and bypass surgery are life-saving procedures that have added years to the lives of many, they are not procedures that most people would like to have done. This is because they are costly, painful, and risky. They don't address the cause of the disease either, yet CSA does. Unfortunately, many people suffering from heart problems view these procedures as the only options. I am now offering you another option: CSA rich collagen type II.

We know that, although genetics play a major role, most heart problems can be avoided through proper diet and exercise. With the availability of treatments like CSA rich collagen type II supplements, there are more options available than most people think.

The problem arises when people have to make the biggest change, a change in lifestyle. A recent television program depicted a man that was facing health problems struggling with his diet. He tried to change, but had become so accustomed to eating fattening, greasy food that he could not get used to the idea of eating fruits and vegetables and other foods that are high in fiber and low in fat and cholesterol.

I know of other people that are set in their ways and refuse to change their diet, or even drink enough water, even though it causes irregularity so severe that medical attention is required. A personal friend told me of his grandmother and the health problems she has had due to her dietary and lifestyle choices. She has been overweight for as long as he can remember, and a few years ago attempted to lose some weight and improve her health. She was starting to make some progress and able to enjoy once more some of the activities that she loved, but decided to give up, since she felt that it was not worth sacrificing the pleasure of eating whatever she wanted to in order to have better health.

Perhaps if she would have stuck to her diet and continued to work towards better health she would not have just had a balloon angioplasty and a valve replacement. Certainly it is worth the sacrifice to make the lifestyle changes necessary to have better health. And with supplements like chondroitin sulfate A rich collagen type II available to help reduce or reverse some of the effects of circulatory disorders, it is a battle that can be won. Remember choice not chance determines your destiny.

Product References		
Brand Name	**Company Name**	**Capsule/ Bottle**
MaxiLIFE Chicken Collagen Type II	Twin Laboratories, Inc. 2120 Smithtown Avenue Ronkonkoma, NY 11779 Tel: (516) 467-3140 http://www.twinlab.com	500mg/30 500mg/60 finished product
Collagen Type II	Natrol, Inc. 21411 Prairie Street Chatsworth, CA 91311 Tel: (800) 326-1520 http://www.natrol.com	500mg/30 500mg/60 finished product
CellRenew	BioCell Technology Tel: (714) 476-3786 (Patent Pending)	Powder, raw material supplier

Product References (cont.)

Brand Name	Company Name	Capsule/ Bottle
CellRenew	Applied Health Solutions Tel: (888) 922-9009 http://appliedhealth.com	500mg/120 finished product
ImmuCell™	Molecule 2000, LLC Tel: (800) 346-2922 http://choicemall.com/molecule2000	500mg/120 finished product
MaxCTII™	Life Source Tel: (800) 886-5415	500mg/120 finished product
Arthenol™ Arthenol Gold™	Health Logics Laboratories, Inc. 675 Fairview Drive #246 Carson City, NV 89701 Tel: (714) 237-1372	500mg/120 500mg/60
ImmuCell™	L & H Vitamins, Inc. Tel: (800) 221-1152	500mg/120 finished product
Colla-Cell II	Power Laboratories, Inc. 12802 Loma Rica Drive #M Grass Valley, CA 95945 Tel: (800) 748-5619	500mg/120
Colla-Cell II ImmuCell™	Nature's Creations 5713 N. Pershing Ave., Ste. C2 Stockton, CA 95207 Tel: (888) 261-1629 Fax: (209) 952-8910 http://www.naturescreations1.com	500mg/120

Alternative Medical Clinic

For more information regarding the alternative medical clinic located in Reno, Nevada, call (800) 552-8885 for free information.

References

1 Bollet, A.J., "Stimulation of Protein-Chondroitin Sulfate Synthesis by Normal and Osteoarthritic Articular Cartilage, *Arthritis and Rheumatism*, vol. 11:663, 1968.

2 Trentham, D.E. et al. *Science*, 1993; 261:1727-1730.

3 Weiss, R. "Genetics to Arthritics: A Gene's The Rub" *Science News* 138:148, 1990.

4 Stehlin, D. "How To Take Your Medicine - Non Steroidal Anti-Inflammatory Drugs" *FDA Consumer*, pp. 33-34, June 1990.

5 Tapadinhas, M.J., Rivera, I.C., and Bignamini, A. A. "Oral Glucosamine Sulphate in the Management of Arthrosis: Report on a Multicentre Open Investigation in Portugal." *Pharmatherapeutica*, 3(3):147-168, 1982.

6 D'Ambrosio, E., et al. "Glucosamine Sulfate: A Controlled Clinical Investigation in Arthrosis." Pharmatherapeutica 2(8):504+, 1981.

7 Dovanti, A., Bignamini, A. A., and Rovati, A. L. "Therapeutic Activity of Oral Glucosamine Sulphate in Osteoarthrosis: A Placebo-Controlled, Double-Blind Investigation." *Clinical Therapeutics* 3(4):266-272, 1980.

8 Pujalte, J.M., Llavore, E.P., and Ylescupidez, E.R. "Double-blind Clinical Evaluation of Oral Glucosamine Sulphate in the Basic Treatment of Osteoarthrosis." *Current Medical Research and Opinion* 7(2):110-114, 1980.

9 Vajaradul, Y. "Double-blind Clinical Evaluation of Intra-articular Glucosamine in Outpatients with Gonarthrosis." *Clinical Therapeutics* 3(5):260+, 1980.

10 Prudden, J.F., and Balassa, L. L. "The Biological Activity of Bovine Cartilage Preparations." *Seminars on Arthritis and Rheumatism* 3(4):287+, 1974.

11 Oliviero. U., et al. "Effects of the Treatment with Matrix on Elderly People with Chronic Articular Degeneration." *Drugs in Experimental and Clinical Research* 17(1):45-51, 1991.

12 Mazieres, B., et al. "Le Chondroitin Sulfate Dayns le Traitement de la Gonarthrose et de la Coxarthrose." *Rev. Rheum. Mal Osteoartic* 59(7-8):466-472, 1992.

13 Trentham, D.E. et al. *Science*, 1993; 261:1727-1730.

14 Barinaga, M. *Science*, 1993; 261:1669-1670.

15 Aigner, T., S. T.-Oss, H., Weseloh, G.; Zeiler, G., vonder Mark, K., "Activa-

tion of Collagen Type II Expression in Osteo Arthritic and Rheumatoid Cartilage" Clinical Research Unit for Rheumatology, University Erlangen-N-Urnberg, Federal Republic of Germany. *Virchows Arch B. Cell. Pathol. Incl. Mol. Pathol.*, 1992, 62:6,337-45.

[16] Barnett, M.L., Combitchi, D., Trentham, D. E., "A Pilot Trial of Oral Type II Collagen in The Treatment of Juvenile Rheumatoid Arthritis," *Arthritis Rheum.*, 1996, April;39(4):623-8.

[17] Miyahara, H., Myers, L.K., Rosloniec, E.F., Brand, D.D., Seyer, J.M., Stuart, J.M., Kang, A.H., "Identification and Characterization of a Major Tolerogenic T-Cell Epitope of Type II Collagen that Suppresses Arthritis in B10 R111 Mice.' *Immunology*, 1995, September 86(1):110-5.

[18] Osborne, A.C., Carter, S.D., May, S.A., Bennett, D. "Anti-Collagen Antibodies and Immune Complexes in Equine Joint Diseases," *Vet-Immuno-Immunopathol*, 1995, March 45(1-2)19-30.

[19] Diab, M. "The Role of Type IX Collagen in Osteoarthritis and Rheumatoid Arthritis." *Orthop-Rev.* 1993, February 22(2):165-70.

[20] Myers, L.K., et al. "T-cell Epitopes of Type II Collagen That Regulate Murine Collagen-Induced Arthritis" *Journal of Immunology* 1993, July 1; 151(1):500-5.

[21] Das,U.N., "Interactions Between Essential Fatty Acids, Eicosanoids, Cytokines, Growth Factors, and Free Radicals: Relevance to New Therapeutic Strategies in Rheumatoid Arthritis and Other Collagen Vascular Diseases." *Prostaglandins-Leukot-Essent Fatty-Acids*, 1991 December;44(4):201-10.

[22] Williams, R.O., Mason, L.J., Feldmann, M., Maini, R.N., "Synergy Between Anti-CD4 and Anti-Tumor Neucrosis Factor in the Amelioration of Established Collagen-Induced Arthritis." *Proc-Nat-Acad-Sci-USA.* 1994, March 29; 91(7):2762-6.

[23] Thompson, H.S., Harper, N., Beavan, D. J., Staines, N.A., "Suppression of Collagen-Induced Arthritis by Oral Administration of Type II Collagen: Changes in Immune and Arthritic Responses by Mediated by Active Proliferal Suppresion" *Auto Immunity* 1993, 16(3):189-99.

[24] Yoshino, S. "Oral Administration of Type II Collagen Suppresses Nonspecifically Induced Chronic Arthritis in Rats" *Biomed-Pharmacother.* 1996; 50(1):24-8.

[25] Rowley,N.J., Cook, A.D., Mackay, I.R., Teuber, S.S., Gershwin, M.E. "Comparative Epitope Mapping of Antibodies to Collagen in Women with Silicone Breast Implants, Systemic Lupus Erythematosis, and Rheumatoid Arthritis." *Curr-Top-Microbiol-Immunol* 1996; 210:307-16.

[26] Naim, J.O., et al. "Induction of Type II Collagen Arthritis in the D.A. Rat using Silicon Gels and Oils as Adjuvant" *Journal of Auto Immunology* 1995, October, 8(5):571-61.

[27] Yoshino, S., "Downregulation of Silicone-Induced Chronic Arthritis by Gastric Administration of Type II Collagen" *Immunopharmacology* 1995, November 31(1):103-8.

[28] Yoshino, K., et al. "Antibodies of Type II Collagen and Immune Com-

plexes in Menier's Disease" *Acta-Otolaryngol-Supplement-Stockh* 1996; 522:79-85.

[29] Thompson, S.J., et al., "Prevention of Pristane-Induced Arthritis by the Oral Administration of Type II Collagen." *Immunology*, 1993, May; 79(1):152-7.

[30] Conte, A. Volpi, N., Palmieri, L., Bahous, I., and Ronca, G., "Biochemical and Pharmacotinetic Aspects of Oral Treatment with Chondroitin Sulfate." *Arzneim-Forsch / Drug Research* 45(11), Nr8(1995).

[31] Murata, K.; Yoshima, Y., et al. "Clinical and experimental studies on mucopolysaccharides, Chapter in Biochemistry and Medicine of Mucoploysaccharides, ed. by F. Egami and Y. Oshima. Published by Research Assoc. of Mucopolysaccharides, Tokyo, Japan. 1962, p. 259.

[32] Fischer, G. and Boedecker, C. Liepigs, Ann. Chem. 117:111/1861.

[33] Virchow, R. Gesammelter abhundiungen zur wissenschaftilchen (Frankfurt, Meidinger) 492, 1889.

[34] Morner, C.T. Skand. Arch. F. Physiol. 1:210, 1889.

[35] Metchnikoff, E. Bulletinde L'institut Pasteur, 7(13):545, 1909.

[36] Meyer, K. Cold Spring Harbor Symposia Quant. Biol. 6:91.

[37] Morrison, L.M., Quilligan, J.J., Jr., Murata, K., Schjeide, O.A., Freeman, L.., Ershoff, B.H., "Treatment of atherosclerosis with acid mucopolysaccharides," *Exper. Med & Surg.* 25:61. 1967

[38] Prudden, J. and Balassa, "The Biological Activity of Bovine Cartilage Preparations." *Sem. Arth. Rheum.* 3(4):287, 1974.

[39] Loeren, W. and Morrison, L., Connect. Tissue Res.1:165.

[40] Schiller, S., "The isolation of chondroitin sulfuric acid from normal human plasma, *Biochem. & Biophys. Acta* 28:413, 1958.

[41] Murata, K. Circulation 38:4, 1969.

[42] Murata, K., "Inhibitory effects of chondroitin polysulfate on lipemia and atherosclerosis in connection with its anticoagulant activity." *Naturwissenschaften* 49:1.

[43] Kaplan, D. and Meyer, K. Proc. Soc. Exp. Biol. Med. 105:78.

[44] Morrison, L.M., Schjeide, O.A., Quilligan, J.J., Jr., Freeman,L., and Murata, K., "Metabolic parameters of the growth-stimulating effect of chondroitin sulfate A in tissue cultures," *Proc. Soc. Exper. Biol & Med.* 119:618, 1965.

[45] Ibid.

[46] Morrison, L. M., Bajwa, G. S., Rucker, P.G., and Ershoff, B. H., "Antithrombogenic effects of chondroitin sulfate A in rats, rabbits and dogs, (abstract), *Am. J. Gerontol.* 17, 913, 1968.

[47] Morrison, L. M., Rucker, P. G., and Ershoff, B. H., "Prolongation of thrombus-formation time in rabbits given chondroitin sulfate." *A. J. Atheroscler. Res.* July, 1968.

[48] Morrison, L. M., Murata, K., Quilligan, J. J., Jr., Schjeide, O. A., Freeman, L., Bajwa, G. S., Bernick, S., Patek, P., Rucker, P., Dunn, O. J., Ershoff, B. H., "The prevention of coronary arteriosclerotic heart disease with chondroitin sulfate A, (abstract) *Circulation* 38:4, 1968.

[49] Morrison, L.M., Schjeide, O.A., Quilligan, J. J., Jr., Freeman, L., and Holeman, R., "Effects of acid mucopolysaccharides on growth rates and constituent lipids of tissue cultures, *Proc. Soc Exper. Biol. Med* 113:362, 1963.

[50] Morrison, L.M., Enrick, N., "Coronary Heart Disease: Reduction of Death Rate by Chondroitin Sulfate A," Angiology of the *Journal of Vascular Diseases,* Vol. 24, No. 5, May 1973, pp. 269-287. Presented at the college of Angiology Congress, Royal College of Surgeons, June 15, 1972, London England.

[51] Morrison, L.M., "Treatment of coronary arteriosclerotic heart disease with chondroitin sulfate A: Preliminary Report," *Journal of the American Geriatrics Society,* Vol. 16, No. 7, July 1968, p.780.

[52] Murata, K., "Inhibitory effects of chondroitin polysulfate on lipemia and atherosclerosis in connection with its anticoagulant activity." *Naturwissenschaften* 49:1.

[53] Enos, et al., *JAMA* 152:1090

[54] Morrison, L. M., Murata, K., Quilligan, J. J., Jr., Schjeide, O. A., Freeman, L., "Prevention of atherosclerosis in sub-human primates by chondroitin sulfate A." *Circulation Res.* 19:338, 1966.

[55] Bajwa and Morrison, *Specialia,* July 15, 1972:1411.

[56] Morrison, L. M., Schjeide, O. A., Quilligan, J. J., Jr., Freeman, L., Murata, K., "Metabolic parameters of the growth-stimulating effect of chondroitin sulfate A in tissue cultures." *Proc. Soc. Exper. Biol. & Med.* 119:618, 1965.

[57] Morrison, L. M., "Response of Ischemic Heart Disease to Chondroitin Sulfate A." *Journal of the American Geriatrics Society,* 17(10):913, 1969.

[58] Morrison, L. M., Murata, K., Quilligan, J. J., Jr., Schjeide, O. A., Freeman, L., Bajwa, G. S., Bernick, S., Patek, P., Rucker, P., Dunn, O. J., Ershoff, B. H., "The prevention of coronary arteriosclerotic heart disease with chondroitin sulfate A, (abstract) *Circulation* 38:4, 1968.

[59] Morrison, L. M., "Reduction of Ischemic Coronary Heart Disease by Chondroitin Sulfate A." *Angiology* 72(3):165, March 1971.

[60] Morrison, L. M., Rucker, P. G., Dunn, O.J, "Prolongation of Thrombus Formation Time in Angina Pectoris by Chondroitin Sulfate A. *Circulation* Vols. 35 & 36, Supplement II, Oct. 1967.

[61] Edwards, D., "Homeopathic Management of Circulatory Disorders." *American Homeopathy* Vol. 1, June 1987.

Index

cold sores 1
colloidal silver 85, 86, 88, 90
colostrum 61
common cold 12, 59
connective tissue 20, 25, 26, 72, 73, 82, 87, 94, 98
copper 24, 39
corticosteroids 4
crepitus 18, 22
Cytomegalovirus 89

D

deafness 71
diabetes 46, 108
dietary factors 12, 24
diuretics 29
dizziness 71
dosage 29, 36, 40, 46, 49, 75, 76, 78, 98, 103
drug poisoning 71

E

essential fatty acids 63, 69, 90, 92

F

fatigue 41, 42
fever 41, 42, 84, 88
fibrocystic disease 68
flax seed oil 63, 92
food sensitivities 92
fungi 43, 86, 94

G

GALT 45, 46, 59, 60, 65
genetic predisposition 15
glucosamine 1-3, 5, 25-33, 36-38, 40, 49, 78, 79, 81-83
Gonococcal Arthritis 84

H

heart attack 34, 97, 101
heart disease 33, 34, 97
heparin 93
hepatitis 25
HIV 86
homeopathic clinic 68

O

occult bleeding 13
omega-3 fats 24
omega-6 fats 24
oral tolerance 45, 46, 56, 64, 65, 66, 69, 75, 76
osteoarthritis 4, 6, 12, 15-17, 19-25, 29, 30, 31, 34-36, 40, 41,
    56, 57, 63, 75, 76, 78, 82, 92, 93, 95, 98

P

painkillers 9, 13, 56
parasites 43, 87
parvo virus 64
plaque 96, 97, 102, 103
prednisone 4, 15, 25
Primary osteoarthritis 19
Primrose oil 92
proteoglycans 1, 2, 4,-7, 13, 19, 23, 25, 26, 28-31, 33-35, 37, 38, 49,
    61, 78, 79, 81-83, 94, 98
psoriasis 1, 3, 4

R

Relafen 50
Rheumatic Fever 84
rheumatism 41
rheumatoid arthritis 4, 12, 16, 17, 19, 34, 40-43, 45-49, 54-57,
    61-65, 67, 71, 75, 76, 78, 83, 87-90, 92
ringing in the ears 71

S

Salmonellae 88
Secondary osteoarthritis 20
shark 2, 6, 40, 69, 93
Shigillae 88
shingles 1
silicone 66, 67, 68, 69, 70
smoking 95
soluble 6, 7, 48, 63
Spondyloarthropathies 91
streptococcus 84
stroke 34, 97
subchondral bone 19, 22
super oxide dismutase 39, 62
synovial fluid 17, 18, 19, 22, 24, 25, 33, 38, 39, 63, 83

synovial membrane 17, 19, 22, 25
synoviocytes 38
synovitis 41
syphilis 71, 85
Syphilitic Arthritis 85
systemic lupus erythematosus 67

T

testimony 7, 8, 9, 50, 51, 52
TNF 60, 62, 63
toxicity 34, 86, 87, 98, 101, 106
trauma 16, 17, 19, 20, 21, 23, 24, 38, 66, 81
tumor necrosis factor 60, 62

U

ulcers 1, 3, 27, 88, 93
uveitis 46

V

viral infections 1
vomiting 71

W

water on the knee 22
white blood cells 37, 60, 62, 75, 83, 84
wound healing 3, 4, 6

Y

Yersiniae 88
yoga 92